THE WORLD'S EMERGENCY ROOM

THE WORLD'S EMERGENCY ROOM

THE GROWING THREAT TO DOCTORS, NURSES, AND HUMANITARIAN WORKERS

MICHAEL VANROOYEN

St. Martin's Press
New York

www.stmartins.com

Design by Letra Libre, Inc.

Library of Congress Cataloging-in-Publication Data

Names: VanRooyen, Michael J.

Title: The world's emergency room : the growing threat to doctors, nurses, and humanitarian workers / Michael VanRooyen.

Description: New York : St. Martins Press, [2016]

Identifiers: LCCN 2015045264| ISBN 9781250072122 (hardcover) | ISBN 9781466883536 (e-book)

Subjects: LCSH: Hospitals—Emergency services—Security measures. | Medical personnel—Violence against. | Medical emergencies. | Emergency physicians. | Emergency medical personnel. | Violence in hospitals—Prevention. | War—Medical aspects. | War—Relief of sick and wounded. | Medicine, Military.

Classification: LCC RA975.5.E5 V36 2016 | DDC 362.18—dc23

LC record available at http://lccn.loc.gov/2015045264

Our books may be purchased in bulk for promotional, educational, or business use. Please contact your local bookseller or the Macmillan Corporate and Premium Sales Department at 1-800-221-7945, extension 5442, or by e-mail at MacmillanSpecialMarkets@macmillan.com.

First Edition: April 2016

10 9 8 7 6 5 4 3 2 1

For 69196-14710

CONTENTS

*Sixteen pages of black and white photos appear
between pages 102 and 103.*

ACKNOWLEDGMENTS

WORKING IN TWO RAPIDLY CHANGING AND DYNAMIC fields—emergency medicine and humanitarian medicine—has been an uncommon privilege. I have been very fortunate to have been guided by mentors, supported by colleagues, and grounded by students and patients. The list of those to thank for their help along the way is too numerous to recount here, but there are a number who should be specifically mentioned, particularly those who provided the right nudge at the right time.

First, of course, is my wife, Julie, and our children, Alexandra, Jack, and Isabella, who provide the emotional respite from the pressures of this work and create an energetic, loving, entertaining, and stabilizing force that brings me ever back to reality. They create balance and normalcy that has been the key to staying in this field for the long haul.

The process of writing a book of personal accounts would have been somewhat disconcerting without the encouragement and reassurance of my editors. Thanks to Pete Beatty, for his clear literary advice and deft editing, and to Jessica Papin, my perpetually positive agent. Thanks to Ben, Courtney, Negeen, and many others for reading through early drafts, and a second thank-you to Julie and Alexandra, who provided smart, thoughtful edits and kept me from rambling.

I have had many mentors in the field who have blazed a trail into this new discipline and who remain thoughtful, brilliant, and inspiring. Kenney Isaacs, Jennifer Leaning, Skip Burkle, Charlie Clements, Peter Walker, Gilbert Burnham, Ron Waldman, Claude Bruderlein, Gabe Kelen, and Ron Walls: you have all encouraged and challenged me to think more creatively and to work harder for the things that really matter.

My faculty and staff at the Harvard Humanitarian Initiative (HHI) are among the most imaginative thinkers in this nascent field of humanitarian studies. Negeen Darani, Enzo Bollettino, Susan Tannehill, and the whole HHI team have been an inspiring reminder of the creativity and courage that exists in this field. Special mention to Jocelyn Kelly, Patrick Vinck, Phuong Pham, Stephanie Kayden, and Hilarie Cranmer for your audacity and resourcefulness. You have all blazed new trails in our field and created a spirit of innovation at HHI that is truly unique. A shout-out also to the Signal Team, the Women in War Program, and the "Child Soldiers of Wayland" for their intimidating presence at our simulations and for the reminder they provide to adults to never underestimate a child soldier.

In a challenging funding environment, a few key supporters have made a tremendous impact on the growth of HHI and allowed us a unique measure of creativity. My deep appreciation goes to Jonathan and Jeannie Lavine who have become both friends and foundational supporters. Fred Weintz and the entire Weintz family were among the very first who invested in HHI when it was simply an idea, and they have helped us move along at every stage. Kristin Mugford, Dom and

Molly Ferrante, Kent Walker and Diana Walsh, Mary Zeintz, Susan Plum, and many others have stepped forward at what seemed to be the most crucial times to provide us the support we needed to grow and flourish. Thanks also to the leadership at the Harvard T. H. Chan School of Public Health, to Michael Voligny and the development team, and to the University's Office of the Provost for your tremendous support of HHI as a new, and sometimes quite unconventional, venture at Harvard.

My thanks also to my colleagues from the many international NGOs and UN agencies that make up the humanitarian community. Responding effectively to the next catastrophe requires organizations that can constantly rethink the way they operate and adapt to the new realities of international aid. In this book, for the sake of brevity, I have oversimplified the humanitarian architecture and the evolving policies that guide global humanitarian aid, but have hopefully emphasized my respect and admiration for the agencies that do the real, hard work.

Finally, for those of us who have worked in the field, we know that our efforts as humanitarian physicians are only a small part of the dedicated efforts of local physicians, nurses, and aid workers who struggle in incredibly tough conditions, risking their lives and livelihoods for their patients. For these caregivers there is no passport to safety. It is with deep respect and humility that I have been able to work alongside you as a colleague.

THE WORLD'S EMERGENCY ROOM

INTRODUCTION

AT A SIGNAL FROM THE MAN IN CHARGE, THE YOUNG soldier shoved the muzzle of his AK-47 into my mouth. The oily metal clanked against my teeth. I tried to jerk away, but a soldier standing behind me pushed me back toward the gun. A hand held my head in place. As terrified as I was, I remember thinking that the gunman wouldn't pull the trigger if it meant putting a bullet through his colleague's hand. The first soldier withdrew the muzzle, leaving a taste of oil and dirt in my mouth. I looked downward, avoiding the commander's gaze. The interrogation continued.

For five hours, six Zairian soldiers and government agents surrounded me in a stifling, dimly lit room. Jabbing their fingers into my chest, they asked over and over, in French and broken English, what I was doing in Bunia. It was December 1996. I had flown in from Kigali, Rwanda, the day before on a relief mission, accompanied by a colleague and our pilot. We were responding to urgent calls from Nyankunde Hospital in northeastern Zaire for food and medical supplies. Refugees of the 1994 Rwandan genocide, forced from camps farther south, were flooding the region. The conflict in Rwanda had unleashed what has been termed the "African World War," and Bunia was about to become its epicenter.

Laurent Kabila, the leader of a rebellion in Zaire, was marching toward Kisangani, the provincial capital, scattering the Zairian army as they advanced. The country's national "army"—a disorganized and corrupt militia—fled northward, looting, raping, and killing as they moved from village to village. The Zairian army was now approaching Bunia, a small town in northern Zaire near Nyankunde Hospital. We arrived in Bunia just a few days ahead of their advance, landing at dusk on the small airstrip outside of the town. My friend Ken Isaacs, pilot Mark Brumbelow, and I were brought to a small, dark office near the airstrip. Our passports were confiscated. We were questioned on the spot by a large man flanked by two young guards holding machine guns. "What are you doing here? Who gave you a visa to come? Who are you working for?" We replied that we were from an American nongovernmental organization, bringing a relief shipment to Nyankunde Hospital. As the sun set, it became darker in the small concrete building. With no electricity at the airport, they stopped the interrogation. The authorities confiscated our plane, leaving it on the tarmac, and placed us under house arrest.

The next day, the interrogation began in earnest. The three of us were separated, and I was brought to a warehouse at gunpoint. I sat in a small, dark, uncomfortably hot room with three interrogators in front of me. Standing behind us were three young soldiers in tattered uniforms clutching AK-47s. One of my interrogators leaned forward, a pistol in his hand. He toyed with it throughout the questioning.

"How did you get a visa?" he asked. I explained that ours were the last visas issued by the Zairian embassy in Kigali just before the diplomats evacuated.

"Why are you here?" he asked again. Speaking a mix of French, English, and Lingala, the local language used by the Zairian military, he accused us of spying for the CIA and the US military and of carrying supplies for the rebel militia. He pointed to my black Doc Martens boots and said they were military issue.

"What is your profession? Who do you really work for?"

I told him I was an emergency physician and a civilian. I was sweating through my shirt and wondered if they saw my fear as guilt. They exchanged glances around the room, and again he pointed with his pistol to my boots. He refused to believe I was a civilian physician.

"You're too thin to be a doctor," he scoffed.

I was getting frustrated. "That's ridiculous," I blurted out.

He shoved the barrel of the AK-47 into my mouth.

I quickly apologized, and the questioning continued.

After the interrogation, we spent four days under house arrest, hearing intermittent news reports on a shortwave radio that the Zairian armed forces were coming closer. They were terrorizing villages as they moved toward Bunia, abducting and raping women as they looted each town. The Rwandan-backed Kabila campaign sought to overthrow the Zairian government and had tacit support from the United States. Anyone coming from Rwanda with clear ties to America would be in danger. The government forces were only about 30 miles outside of Bunia, but their convoy was delayed by rain and muddy roads.

Two local physicians bravely stepped forward to help negotiate our release. Dr. Tony Ukete and Dr. Ahuka Ona Longombe, both revered surgeons in Zaire, were well known among the community and the militia holding us. They leveraged their influence on our behalf. In a peculiar irony, my "military" boots were also the key to our release: after we distributed bribes totaling about $7,600 from the cash concealed in their soles, we were allowed to leave. We were forced to sign deportation papers before making our way on the tarmac to the Cessna Caravan, a ten-passenger, single-engine plane commonly used to travel between small airports in East Africa. We were instructed by our captors to fly to Kampala, Uganda, carrying with us an Egyptian arms dealer, but I was concerned that he might be carrying a gun and, once airborne, could force us to fly elsewhere. We finally agreed to take him along, but only after I insisted that we search him for weapons. Having never searched anyone before, I apologized as I patted him down on the airstrip outside the plane. I think he was more nervous than I, and we both were anxious to get out of Bunia. After making sure our Egyptian passenger was indeed unarmed, we boarded the plane and awaited clearance to depart.

Finally, we were airborne. Bunia slowly disappeared from view as we flew over the Zairian countryside. I breathed a sigh of relief as we officially entered Ugandan airspace.

The hospital we had set out to aid did not fare as well. In the months that followed, most of the medical staff were evacuated. Many national staff and patients were killed or forced to flee, and the facility was looted and ransacked. Nyankunde Hospital, a beacon of health care for the entire region, was destroyed.

1

DISCOVERING
HUMANITARIANISM

MUCH OF THE WORLD SEEMS TO BE ON FIRE. THE second decade of the twenty-first century has shown us some of the most complex and dangerous political struggles in recent history. Since it began in 2011, the Syrian Civil War has morphed from a one-country political uprising to a regional conflict that has displaced 9 million civilians and killed over 200,000, many of them through the use of chemical weapons. The rise of the Islamic State of Iraq and Syria (ISIS) has once again pulled the United States into Iraq, where it is providing military intervention to protect civilians and establish a corridor for humanitarian aid. An unprecedented Ebola epidemic in West Africa in 2014 threatened to destabilize the healthcare systems, economies, and governments of Sierra Leone, Liberia, and the rest of West Africa.

The human consequences of conflict and disaster are profound. Today, nearly 60 million people have been displaced from their homes by war or catastrophe, more than at any time since World War II. While such huge numbers can feel abstract, the threats to families and communities are very real and very personal. Refugees live in makeshift shelters and temporary settlements, struggling day by day to survive. They have little food, not enough clean water, and few resources for health care for their children. Rates of malnutrition, diarrhea, and respiratory infection are exponentially higher among refugees than among the population at large. The same is true for violent crimes like rape, abduction, and human trafficking.

Humanitarian aid workers are on the front lines of these conflicts. Aid organizations employ international and local staff to rapidly take the place of systems that have failed because of war or disaster. Aid agencies provide emergency relief—food, water, shelter, security, and health care—to stabilize populations in the midst of a crisis. Humanitarian medicine, the emergency provision of basic health care, serves some of the world's most acutely threatened populations.

The doctors and nurses who work at the front lines of crises, many of them local healthcare providers, save lives in places where normal healthcare systems have broken down. They work in uncontrolled and often-dangerous environments with few resources to keep hospitals open, perform lifesaving surgery, and provide essential medications for people trapped in conflict with nowhere else to turn. They innovate, improvise, and create a "safety net" for a community. These caregivers not only staff, but *build* a global emergency room.

As a humanitarian physician, I've worked in hot spots and conflict areas all around the world. I return from missions abroad and dive right back into busy urban medical centers in Detroit, Chicago, Baltimore, and now at home in Boston, places where emergency room physicians serve as providers of last resort, caring for many who have no regular health care. Throughout the past twenty-five years, I've tried to balance my international work with practicing medicine in urban ERs in the United States. During this time, I have observed several common traits in these two diverse fields.

My patients in Boston are, of course, a world apart from my patients in Rwanda or Sudan. They face different struggles and have profoundly different vulnerabilities. But the systems that serve them have some important similarities. In a humanitarian crisis, nongovernmental organizations (NGOs) like Médecins Sans Frontières (MSF, also known in the English-speaking world as Doctors Without Borders) struggle to provide medical assistance to those who are displaced or threatened. In the emergency departments of our nation, the medical staff stands ready to provide care for anyone, anytime, regardless of ability to pay or the nature of their ailment. The ER serves as a safety net for many in our communities who suffer from acute illness, trauma, or untreated medical problems.

During my years of work abroad, I've found that the international aid community—a web of NGOs, United Nations (UN) agencies, and governmental departments—provides a similar safety net. Conflict and disaster affect many more civilians than soldiers and often lead to high mortality rates, particularly in infants and children. The unchecked spread of preventable infectious diseases like measles and diarrhea drives high death rates in refugee and malnourished populations. War and displacement have predictable and devastating effects on health. In these contexts, humanitarians provide the rapid, large-scale aid that is critical for stabilizing populations and providing the first step toward recovery and resilience. What the emergency room is to Detroit, Chicago, and Baltimore, humanitarian medical relief is to the world's crisis zones.

The problems and threats created by a humanitarian crisis require specialized and nuanced skills that are distinct from those employed in long-term development pursuits like agricultural projects and public health programs. Humanitarian medicine is a unique field with a specific base of knowledge and, much like emergency medicine, requires a specialized skill set. While the actual services delivered by each field are very different, many aspects of their environments are strikingly similar.

Paradoxically, the humanitarians who care for some of the most vulnerable populations in the most hostile settings in the world are often not trained for the job. Most of the world's 450,000 humanitarian aid workers lack any formal training, certification, or professional identity. As the aid community grows and matures, there is an increasing awareness of the importance of professional development and the need for better research and evidence to advance the field. Within the wider aid community, the quality and accountability of aid are major new foci. Humanitarianism must evolve to better face the challenges of ever-more complex humanitarian crises.

I've grown as an ER doctor and as a humanitarian physician simultaneously, at a time when both fields have faced tremendous challenges and seen major improvements. As new crises emerge, our only appropriate response is to adapt and apply lessons we've learned to create new tools to make a better, more efficient relief world. The lives of our patients, and the world's most vulnerable populations, depend upon it.

The seeds for my work were sown early. Like any child, my interests were the product of a unique blend of influences and inspirations. In many ways, my childhood in St. Johns, Michigan, was typically American. But my parents—and their journeys through life—subtly led me toward both medicine and traveling the world. That voyage began with the numbers tattooed on my father's arms.

My earliest impressions of the world outside of small-town Michigan came from my father. Johannes (Joe) VanRooyen was a Dutch immigrant and Holocaust survivor. Like all fathers, he told many stories of his boyhood and growing up. He had a rich library from which to draw, and my brother Rick and I spent many hours hearing about his early life in the Netherlands and the numerous colorful characters in my extended family. But for all the memories my father shared, he spoke little of the most impactful period of his life: his experience with the Dutch Resistance and his imprisonment in Nazi concentration camps.

The Nazi army invaded the Netherlands on May 10, 1940. After a five-day campaign, a brutal occupation began. The German stranglehold on the Netherlands was severe, with the army intent on extracting resources and wealth to feed their war machine and, in the process, starving the country. My father and grandmother buried silverware and other valuables—even his beloved motorcycle—in their garden to prevent them from being looted by the Nazis. At seventeen, unbeknownst to his parents, my father joined the Dutch resistance movement that sought to hide Jews and assist in their escape. He snuck fugitive Jews to the port town of Vlissingen, where boats waited to carry them to England, and aided a downed American pilot trying to reach the border via bicycle (the pilot eventually made it to neutral Spain). "Many times there were narrow escapes," my father later wrote, "but in 1943, I finally got caught."

He was sent to a detention center at Amersfoort, where he was questioned for several weeks. From there he was taken to a crowded boxcar that brought him to another camp, and he eventually ended up in Bergen-Belsen, the infamous Nazi camp located in northern Germany that held tens of thousands of Jews, prisoners of war, and political prisoners. There were no gas chambers at Bergen-Belsen, but over the course of the war, more than 50,000 prisoners would die there, mostly from malnutrition, tuberculosis, or typhus.

Upon arrival at Bergen-Belsen, Joe VanRooyen was registered, hosed off, de-loused, and given the typical striped uniform. Ultimately, during his time in the camps, the number 69196 was tattooed on his left forearm, and 14710 on his right. As a child, I asked my father about the tattoos, about the camps, and about his life before emigration to America. Like many men of his generation, he spoke little about his experiences during World War II. Only rarely, while we were fishing or puttering in his workshop, would he quietly reflect on those times. But he left out the most graphic details of imprisonment. Only gradually, over the course of years, would I learn the horrific, full story of his capture, the starvation and torture prisoners faced in the camps, and the physical and mental abuse he suffered.

After arriving at the camps, my father was put to work at Bamag-Meguin, a factory where steel was shaped and molded for the Nazi war effort. Classified as a political prisoner, he was thought to have information about the resistance movement. Not yet twenty years old, Joe was brought several times from Bergen-Belsen to Alexanderplatz in Berlin to undergo interrogation by the Gestapo in a room deep underground. First Nazi interrogators wound his body in rawhide leather straps soaked in water and laid him on the floor. As the leather slowly dried and contracted, his fingernails were driven into his hands. The pain was excruciating. He was questioned for several days and then returned to his barracks, only to be brought back for questioning again a month later. He recounted the experience in an audio journal later in life:

> A month later, the questioning started again; this time I was strapped in a chair. A hole was drilled in my tooth and a small chain with a winch fastened on that. Every question got a little tap on the winch and after several hours the tooth came out and another one was started. After three days (or was it four or five? I don't remember) they started to drill a hole into the roof of my mouth to hook the chain on. Then I passed out, knowing that this was the end. Somehow, they didn't do much damage to my mouth. How and what happened then, I don't know, but I woke up in my barracks where my roommates took care of me and had washed my face and gave me some warm water to drink.

He had little information that would have been of value to his captors, but saw silence as his only hope: "I could not tell anything because my chance to survive would be gone," he remembered. "I'd become useless to them." He managed to endure the torture, the forced labor, and the near-starvation, and was liberated by Allied troops in April 1945. On the day he was liberated, my five-foot, eight-inch father weighed seventy-eight pounds. Returning to the Netherlands, he found a country ravaged by the war. The mass starvation of the 1944–1945 "Hunger Winter" and the collapse of the economy had left my father's world in tatters. Upon his return, he eagerly dug up the motorcycle that he had buried in the backyard, but found it rusted and rotted away. He struggled with depression, made worse by the failure of a brief business venture. He felt like a stranger in his own hometown and struggled to relate to his family. The economy of postwar Holland was devastated, and he, like many of his generation, looked across the ocean for a chance to start anew. He met and married my mother, Gertrude Breed, a young woman from Haarlem. My parents pinned their hopes for the future on moving to America. On Christmas Eve 1954, they received their long-sought visas.

Joe and Trudy VanRooyen emigrated in 1955, eventually settling in St. Johns, Michigan. Dutch heritage runs deep in that part of the state, but St. Johns could not have been more different from the wartorn Netherlands. Grateful for a fresh start, my father set to work with an immigrant's drive and industriousness, first at a furniture store, then as a shoe salesman, and finally as a cobbler, with his own shoe repair shop. He and my mother were proud to become US citizens, and prouder yet to start their own American family with the birth of my brother Richard in 1957. I was born four years later.

Even though my father was guarded about his wartime experiences, cautious about sharing too much detail and rarely speaking about his captivity, I formed a strong impression of what war meant to ordinary people. I understood that conflict had devastated my father's homeland and nearly killed him. I knew that he was lucky to be alive, and that I was doubly lucky to be here, in America, safe and free. To me, war was never about patriotism, uniforms, and salutes. While I admired the bravery of soldiers and understood the necessity of some conflicts, I never thought war was noble or idealistic; I always saw it as brutal and evil, the most terrible of human endeavors.

My father was immensely proud of his adopted country and of the stable and happy life he and my mother built for their sons. But a decade after their emigration, the foundation of that life was rocked when my thirty-six-year-old mother received a grave medical diagnosis: stage IV metastatic melanoma, the deadliest type of skin cancer. Doctors gave her less than a year to live. I was five years old, and my brother was nine.

She managed to survive for three years, with the help of surgery, chemotherapy, and increasingly long hospitalizations, as the medical system in the 1960s supported extended hospital stays for cancer patients. She spent her days at home trying to create a normal life for us, but I could see her becoming more frail as the disease progressed. Late in her illness, my mother was gone for what seemed like months at a time. In those days, children my age were not allowed in patients' rooms, so I spent countless hours in hospital waiting rooms and parking lots while my father and brother visited her. I can still picture her waving to me from the window of her third-floor hospital room while I waited in the car.

I spent my seventh birthday in the cafeteria of the University Hospital in Ann Arbor. After cake and presents, my father and brother went upstairs to visit my mother while I waited in the hospital cafeteria. My dad had given me a rather unusual gift for my birthday: a world atlas. I sat in that busy cafeteria by myself, poring over maps of Africa, tracing the line of the Congo River and memorizing the names of countries— Sudan, Ethiopia, Tanzania, Kenya—that seemed so exotic and far away. My imagination was already captivated by the television series *Daktari*, about a veterinarian in East Africa, and by stories I'd heard in school about missionaries and military doctors. I sensed there was some greater purpose in working overseas and dreamed about being a doctor in the distant countries that filled the pages of my atlas.

As the months passed, I largely experienced my mother's illness through my father, overhearing his conversations with the doctors and nurses caring for her and the many friends who pitched in to help. He carried on with stoic calm, always telling my brother and me that everything would be all right. But we could sense the strain was taking a toll. Like anyone would, my father struggled to manage my mother's worsening illness and mounting medical bills while taking care of two small children.

My mother had cancer at a time when patients and families didn't question doctors, and doctors rarely involved them in making medical decisions. I knew my father was frustrated by the lack of information, and I remember him going back to her doctors many times to try to understand the next phase of her treatment. I didn't understand what was happening and felt confused by it all. I felt like a burden. I could only stand back, confused, excluded, and helpless, waiting for the next bit of news from my father. And the news only grew worse. On November 16, 1969, my mother died at the age of thirty-nine. She was buried three days later, on my eighth birthday.

My father, brother, and I went on, as families do, with work, school, and life. In time I came to enjoy our bachelor existence. In our single-parent household, I had an unusual degree of independence for a boy my age. I was free to roam our small town on my own, making Tang sandwiches and riding bikes with my friends, exploring the woods, cattle yards, and construction sites around town. But for my father, the life of a widower was a lonely one. While there was always help from our community, he needed companionship. In time he began seeing Carolyn Riley, a close friend of my mother's who had helped our family during her illness. They had reconnected when my father volunteered in the "Big Brothers" program to work with her oldest sons. Their friendship grew, and they fell in love. Three years after my mother's death, they married.

Carolyn had recently divorced an abusive husband and lived in the countryside outside of St. Johns with her eight children, Terry, Fran, Maggie, Pat, Rose, Joyce, Michael (yes, another Michael), and Bill. After the wedding, the nine of them moved into our house, and we became one big, complicated family. Going from a household of three to one of twelve—and suddenly acquiring five sisters, three brothers, and a new mother—was a massive change. My brother and I went from having our own rooms to living in what seemed like a dormitory. Hand-me-downs and powdered milk helped stretch the family budget. An egg timer made sure no one lingered too long in the shower, and labeled poker chips on a board by the door tracked our comings and goings. As we kids reached driving age, seven or eight cars with a cumulative value of about $200 appeared in the yard. We had our share of clashes and minor calamities, but on the whole, our crowded, hectic household thrived. What I had given up in freedom I more than gained in the sense of belonging to a large, loud, and sometimes unruly tribe.

Still, not surprisingly, I looked for ways to get out of the house. The Boy Scouts answered that need for independence. Troop 81 met every Wednesday evening at the Congregational church, and it gave me new friends, new mentors, and a new sense of identity and purpose. I loved learning camping skills and being outdoors, both big parts of scouting. So was public service, and I got a lot of satisfaction out of helping with roadside cleanups, nursing home visits, and city disaster drills. My progress toward Eagle Scout was impeded by, of all things, first-aid training. It was the only merit badge I flunked—twice. It was taught by the chief of police in our town, and I grew nervous and flustered when I was faced with an imaginary medical emergency. CPR class was especially tough, since it seemed, even with a mannequin, to be a matter of life or death.

I finally passed, but I was embarrassed by my shakiness under pressure. I wondered how I would react in a real emergency.

I got a chance to find out the summer I was fourteen, in an experience that set me on a course toward emergency medicine. My troop leader, Chris Cook, had hired me to help on his farm. We plowed fields, cleaned out stalls, baled hay, and cultivated his cornfields. I enjoyed working hard, and I loved spending time on the farm and learning about everything from driving a tractor to fixing the combine. One afternoon, after we had finished hauling a load of creosote-soaked lumber, Chris let me drive the pickup back to his place along a country road. As we drove, we saw smoke ahead and soon came upon a terrible accident. A huge tractor was flipped upside down in the middle of the road, and the terrified driver, a teenager not much older than I, was pinned beneath it, folded in half in a puddle of vomit and red transmission fluid (which I thought was blood) that dripped from the hissing engine. While Chris raced off in the truck to get help, I knelt beside the young victim.

"I don't want to die," he said in a shaky voice.

"You're going to be OK," I told him, having no idea whether that was true. I was nearly as terrified as the injured boy, but I fixed my eyes on his, held his hand, and reassured him that help was on the way. A small army of volunteer firefighters and ambulance crews arrived quickly, with sirens blaring and red lights flashing. I was struck by how calm and controlled these local first responders were. There must have been more than thirty of them, but they worked efficiently. They let me stay with the boy while the firefighters hooked up a heavy-duty wrecker to the tractor. The two-ton machine groaned and creaked, dripping hot oil on the pavement, as it was lifted off him. Then the emergency medical technicians (EMTs) rushed in and carefully but swiftly bore him away to the hospital.

I later learned that the young driver had fractured his pelvis and broken his back, but he eventually recovered fully. I was transformed by what I had seen. I was in awe of the way the volunteers had responded so quickly and acted so coolly to save a life. They were everything I wanted to be: calm, confident, and prepared in the face of a real crisis. They were the ones that people turned to for help, and I wanted to be one of them.

2

FIRST STEPS

MY EXPERIENCES AS A TEENAGER IN ST. JOHNS WILL be familiar to anyone who attended a public high school in a small town: friends, football games, schoolwork, and clubs. Coming from a large family with limited means meant that me and most of my siblings had part-time jobs. I worked with my father in his shoe store and learned some basic shoe-repair skills. I also worked for several years at Parr's Pharmacy, where I was a stock boy. After work, I studied. I was a solid student but probably too involved with extracurricular activities to excel academically. Instead, I thrived by being busy. School government, drama performances, and work filled my days and helped make me independent.

In 1978, during my junior year, my father suffered a near-fatal heart attack. He suddenly developed chest pain while at home, and my stepmother Carolyn took him straight to the emergency room at our small local hospital. With just a few beds, the ER at Clinton Memorial Hospital was not exactly a real emergency room. Staffed by a single nurse, the treatment offered there was generally limited to cuts, falls, and minor emergencies. My father was having a massive myocardial infarction.

In 1962, about sixteen years before my father's heart attack, cardiologist Bernard Lown of Brigham and Women's Hospital and Harvard Medical School introduced the first direct-current external cardiac defibrillator. Over the next several years, the new device was tested and brought into production, making its way to ambulances and emergency rooms. The defibrillator eventually became a standard feature of emergency departments all over the country. Even the tiny ER at Clinton Memorial Hospital had acquired one.

When my father went into ventricular fibrillation, his heart stopped beating, and the nurse in the ER sprang quickly into action, placing the external defibrillator's electrodes on his chest. The device "shocked" him from cardiac arrest to a normal heart rhythm. My father regained a pulse. He would eventually recover completely, walking out of the hospital and back to his family. More than thirty years later, as an ER physician at Brigham and Women's Hospital, I attended a lecture in honor of Dr. Lown at Harvard Medical School. After the lecture, I made my way to the front of the auditorium and thanked him.

After his heart attack, my father needed to recuperate for a few months. He could not run his shoe-repair business—but the store was the sole source of income for our family and could not close. My stepmother could manage the store sales, but someone needed to keep the repair business going. So, in the fall of my junior year, I left school early each day to help run the store. My father recovered in a few months, as did the business, and I returned to the life of a full-time student. The next year, in 1980, my sister Joyce and I graduated in the same class at high school—and we were not alone. Without our knowing it, my father and stepmother, neither of whom had graduated high school, had been attending night school to obtain their GED certifications just in time to graduate alongside Joyce and me.

Choosing a college was a matter of financial aid. The road to a career in medicine included four years of college, four years of medical school, and another three or four years of residency. I had few savings and would not be able to attend an undergraduate institution unless I could receive scholarships and enroll in a work-study program. I was fortunate to be accepted to a pre-medical program at Michigan State University, and scholarships, grants, and work-study allowed me to graduate from college debt-free. I began my studies at Lyman Briggs, a small residential college within Michigan State University, in the fall of 1980. Lyman Briggs was a perfect program for me, offering smaller classes and professors who got to know me well and who provided both instruction and career advice. The pre-med curriculum was intense. Courses like organic chemistry, physics, and biochemistry favored students who were organized and disciplined. I had to learn to be both, and neither came easily. Nevertheless, the demanding program prepared me well for medical school.

My interview for medical school at Wayne State University in Detroit proved an accidental early milestone in my career at the intersection of emergency medicine and public health. I learned just before the interview that my interviewer was an epidemiologist-physician: a clinician who saw patients, but also conducted research on epidemic diseases in large populations. Just before our appointment, I found the medical library and looked up one of his articles on malaria transmission. The first question he asked as we sat down for our interview was why the field of epidemiology was important. We talked about the emerging AIDS pandemic, about how malaria was still the single biggest killer in the world, and about poverty's status as the most important factor driving lower life expectancy and social inequity. From this one-hour interview, I not only gained admission to medical school but for the first time realized the important interplay between poverty and poor health, and how academic physicians could address social problems on a global scale.

Like any first-year medical student, I had to adjust. Pre-med had been a challenge, but medical school was all consuming. During my first two years, courses in anatomy, pathology, physiology, and pharmacology kept me glued to my texts (and cadavers) with little time to think about the future. The amount of information to digest was immense, and the pace was relentless. Wayne State presented the additional challenge of living and studying in Detroit. In 1984, the city was already well into the economic decline that would culminate in bankruptcy three decades later. The neighborhoods around the medical school were impoverished and violent. The vulnerabilities to which poverty exposed the population were evident at every corner of the city, and there were endless social and medical needs. My studies at Wayne State also brought me into contact with some of the most dedicated doctors I've ever seen, and many others who served the poor of the city with a clear sense of purpose. These individuals ran inner-city practices, staffed free clinics, and managed drug rehab programs. A notion grew in me that the privilege of being a physician bore the responsibility of service—but I wasn't yet sure where that realization would lead me.

After the first two years of basic medical science, I began clinical rotations. Treating real patients was a welcome relief from the endless studying. I immediately began to consider what my medical specialty might be and how I could combine medicine with my desire to work internationally. I spent long hours in the library reading about tropical medicine and public health programs. I paid close attention to news about global health and developed a particular interest in disasters and conflict. I also talked often with my father about my studies. As he grew older, he became more candid about his wartime experiences and the suffering he had lived through in the wake of conflict. I began thinking more about how I could work abroad and apply my medical training to some larger global purpose, but I wasn't sure how to begin.

Even while buried in my medical studies, I continued to be drawn to the global political news of the day. In the 1980s, war, disaster, and revolution seemed to be reshaping the world. In April 1985, a coup re-ignited a dormant civil war in Sudan. A year later, an explosion and fire at the Chernobyl nuclear power plant in Ukraine released a massive plume of radioactive material into the atmosphere over the western Soviet Union and northern Europe. Battles raged between Soviet troops and the Mujahedeen in Afghanistan. These events and others drove the number of refugees and internally displaced people to triple between 1985 and 1990, from 15 million to nearly 45 million, more than at any time since World War II.

More than 2.5 million of these refugees were in the Horn of Africa, where drought and famine had compounded the effects of political upheaval and civil war for the people of Sudan, Somalia, and especially Ethiopia. A 1984 BBC news report on the "biblical famine" in Ethiopia, which ultimately claimed some 1 million lives, captured the world's attention.[1] Images of skeletally thin children dying in their mothers' arms prompted an unprecedented outpouring of government and private aid. The famine resulted from more than a lack of food; it also stemmed from political insecurity, lack of food production, and economic collapse, which led to desperate food shortages, skyrocketing prices, and, finally, migration and starvation. In July 1985, as a medical student, I was one of 1.5 billion people who watched Bob Geldof's epic Live Aid concerts for Ethiopian famine relief. The transatlantic event featured the biggest names in music and raised tens of millions of dollars for the relief effort. It put international humanitarian relief in the spotlight like never before and projected an image of aid workers as selfless saviors.

I continued to follow the news reports from Ethiopia, as well as those from Afghanistan, Ukraine, and other hot spots, viewing them through the lens of my father's World War II experiences. I felt a powerful empathy for the victims of famine, war, and disaster, and was drawn to help. Humanitarian aid seemed like the perfect fit for a physician with an interest in global crises, but the aid world seemed so foreign and far away. The question was how to get from here to there. Medical school challenged and fascinated me on a daily basis, but I wasn't seeing the connection between what I was learning in the hospital and what I wanted to do in the field. I still had years of training to complete, and I was getting impatient. In the meantime, I joined the activist group International Physicians for the Prevention of Nuclear War (co-founded by the same Dr. Bernard Lown who invented the defibrillator) and volunteered at homeless shelters, but I still didn't feel as though I had moved any further along my path. I began to wonder if I belonged in a different profession. Considering the possibility that high-tech Western medicine was the wrong route for me, I contemplated a career in public health or even international diplomacy.

Just as I began my junior year, I read *Witness to War: An American Doctor in El Salvador* by Dr. Charles Clements, published in 1984. As an Air Force pilot, Clements had flown more than fifty missions during the Vietnam War, including bombing runs over officially neutral Cambodia. After nine months of active duty, he concluded that America's secret war in Cambodia was immoral and refused to fly further missions. Deemed mentally unfit and discharged by the Air Force, Clements became a Quaker and went to medical school. He also became a human rights activist. In the early 1980s, alarmed by growing US support for the repressive military government in El Salvador, Clements spent a year behind rebel lines there caring for victims of the civil war that left-wing guerilla groups were waging against the government.

Witness to War aimed to shed light on the brutality the United States was underwriting through its anti-communist Reagan Doctrine in Central America. "I've been called a communist," Clements said at the time. "I'm not. I'm a humanist and I'm involved in El Salvador because our government is responsible for much of the violence. The US is sounding increasingly as it did in Vietnam 15 years ago, and I'm very aware of what that led to."[2] His path—combining care for victims of conflict with the use of medicine as a vehicle for political change—was a revelation to me. Years later, I would come to work with Charlie, and today I am honored to call him a friend and colleague at Harvard, where he was the executive director of the Carr Center for Human Rights Policy. Charlie's book convinced me that medicine was where I belonged; I just needed a different kind of medicine. I had to find a way to make my medical practice adaptable and transportable from US inner cities to conflict zones around the world. More immediately, I needed to figure out what type of training would equip me for such a journey.

During their third and fourth years medical students rotate through an array of specialties, spending several weeks to a few months learning from doctors in internal medicine, pediatrics, surgery, obstetrics and gynecology, and psychiatry. Many students find their way into a particular field through an inspiring clinical rotation, and I was one of them. My first day at Detroit Receiving Hospital's emergency department brought salvation from months of indecision.

The huge inner-city ER was beyond busy; it was pandemonium. In 1986, the use of crack cocaine had reached epidemic proportions, and so had violent clashes between drug dealers vying for control of the lucrative trade. Detroit was a major battleground in the crack wars, and the ER at Detroit Receiving was like a combat hospital. Patients on stretchers lined the hallways. Treatment rooms were packed. Ambulances queued up outside, full of still more ill and injured people. The medical staff swarmed around, seemingly in chaos. Yet everyone knew exactly what he or she was doing. Each new gunshot victim or cardiac arrest elicited a rapid response from the staff. No matter how busy they were, the team at Detroit Receiving took the next case, and the next. The energy, intensity, and sheer unpredictability of the ER drew me in immediately.

Upon my arrival on rotation, the senior resident, Brian O'Neil, spotted me and introduced himself: "Welcome to the ER. Let's get you started." He was young, confident, and energetic. He moved through the ER effortlessly, managing the care of a dozen patients. He seemed to know everything. Quick-witted and decisive, he was everything I imagined an ER doctor should be. O'Neil was also an excellent mentor. He gave me a greater degree of responsibility and autonomy than I had had on other rotations. The freedom was exhilarating. I splinted fractures, sutured lacerations, and performed CPR during codes. The ER felt different from any other medical environment I'd been in, and I loved being part of a team in which doctors, residents, nurses, and techs all worked together and all depended on each other. Maybe growing up with nine brothers and sisters made the swarm feel like home. The ER brought together everything I loved about medicine.

I had arrived at a turning point for the hospital. Detroit Receiving was one of the first emergency medicine training programs in the United States. Their postgraduate emergency medicine training program was launched in 1976, three years before emergency medicine was recognized by the American Board of Medical Specialties. Even into the 1980s, most American emergency rooms were crowded, poorly equipped places staffed by interns and medical students. Young doctors, with no formal training in trauma or resuscitation and with little oversight from senior physicians, treated gunshot wounds, head injuries, heart attacks, and strokes. In other words, the least experienced providers were handling the most acute and complex cases, and to the peril of their patients.

O'Neil, who today chairs Wayne State's Department of Emergency Medicine, helped me see that this brand-new field was aching for development and innovation. He and his colleagues were not only clinicians, but also scientists, conducting both lab-based and clinical research on cardiac resuscitation, brain injury, toxicology, and pre-hospital ambulance care. By the time my four-week rotation was over, I knew that emergency medicine was where I belonged. I had found my specialty. But I still needed to figure out how to apply it to public health globally.

At the end of my fourth and final year of medical school, I completed my required rotations early and spent several months traveling abroad, searching for connections between medicine and humanitarian aid. I wanted to explore the field of disaster relief to understand how I could get involved. My plan was vague and naïve. I would work with a disaster relief organization in India, interview leaders in the aid community in Geneva, and follow Charlie Clements's footsteps to El Salvador. I had no real financing, but I was awarded a cultural scholarship through an El Salvador community center in Detroit to create a series of paintings for an exhibit on the El Salvadoran civil war. I had painted for several years in oil, acrylic, and watercolor, and embraced this unique opportunity to apply my interest in art to this rather unusual new setting. The scholarship funded my flights, and I patched together the difference by arranging housing with friends, families, and generous contacts.

I traveled first to Delhi, where I was to spend several weeks working at the cardiology service at the All India Institute for Medical Sciences (AIIMS), a famous public hospital in New Delhi, the home of world-renowned experts in infectious diseases, surgery, and internal medicine. Because resources were so limited, physicians at AIIMS developed sophisticated physical diagnostic skills instead of sending patients for testing. I planned to work with the cardiology service at AIIMS for several weeks and then to work with the Indian Red Cross.

When I arrived in India, my first impression was that it was exotic and fascinating. The author Rudyard Kipling probably said it best when he remarked that "the first condition of understanding a foreign country is to smell it." India was too much of everything. The crush of people was like nothing I had ever seen, with shops and people everywhere. There were cows walking in the streets, vendors at every turn, and motorized rickshaws filling every space of road. The pace was frenzied, the sights were strange, and the food was fragrant and fabulous.

As a first-time global traveler, I felt indestructible. I haggled over the price of a trinket, chewed through betel nut leaves, and sat on the floor of a roadside restaurant, eating curry and drinking milk tea. I wanted to taste all of it, experience all of it. It turned out that "all of it" was a bit too much. As I walked into my first morning of cardiology rounds at AIIMS the day after my arrival, I broke into a sweat, felt a wave of nausea, and ran down the hall in search of a toilet, where I stayed for hours, fighting a debilitating bout of "Delhi Belly." After sheepishly sneaking out of the hospital, having missed rounds entirely, I finally made my way back to my host family. I disappeared for most of the week, retreating to my small room and trying to stop vomiting long enough to hold down some water. I emerged with a deep respect for food poisoning and was filled with dread at the mere mention of "curry." Embarrassed that I had become so ill immediately upon arriving in India, I felt like a novice traveler. It was one of many early lessons in travel health and, in the larger sense, in humility.

When I was well enough to resume work, it was as a volunteer with the Indian Red Cross in Delhi, which was then assisting several thousand people who had been forced from their homes by flooding outside of Delhi a few weeks before my arrival. It hardly resembled the major disasters I had seen on television, but it did require the most basic kind of community health work to assist those people who had lost everything. We would meet at the office or at one of the warehouses, where we would load several large lorries full of food, blankets, buckets, and soap, and drive as close as we could get to the crowded, muddy slums. Hundreds of local volunteers would help us unload and distribute materials to people who had been forced out of their small homes by the flood. Thousands of people lined up to collect buckets full of supplies from the back of the truck. The scene of so many people, ankle deep in mud, pushing to get closer was overwhelming. But after the first hours, I became accustomed to the press of bodies and began to feel like part of this bigger effort. While the situation felt desperate and chaotic, it was infused with a spirit of kindness that impressed me greatly. We spent the rest of the week loading supplies, driving them out to the sodden slums, and helping people dig through the rubbish to recover what few goods they had. The poverty was crushing, but the prevailing emotion, improbably, seemed to be that of hope. Everyone, from the Indian Red Cross leaders to the local volunteers, was gentle and generous. This was not large-scale humanitarianism, but relief by the community, for the community. And it worked.

Because of Charlie Clements's book, I wanted to go to El Salvador, which in 1988 was two-thirds of the way through its twelve-year civil war. Clements's voice was one of many raised against the Reagan administration's support for President José Napoleón Duarte and his brutal junta. The conflict would kill more than 75,000 Salvadorans and displace another 1 million—nearly 20 percent of the population—before peace accords were signed in 1992. Compounding this, in 1986 the small Central American nation had been devastated by an earthquake that had left 1,500 people dead, 10,000 injured, and 200,000 homeless in and around the capital city of San Salvador.

I wanted to see for myself what war was doing to the civilian population, and so I volunteered in Santa Ana, El Salvador's second-largest city, with a group of Maryknoll priests who embraced liberation theology, a doctrine that sees resisting unjust economic, social, and political conditions as part of the Christian mission. Catholic priests and nuns had paid a heavy price for their advocacy on behalf of El Salvador's poor and disenfranchised. In March 1980 Archbishop Óscar Romero, a high-profile critic of the junta, was shot dead while celebrating Mass. Eight months later, three American nuns and a lay missionary were abducted, raped, and murdered. All of these killings were the work of government forces.

But the five priests with whom I lived and volunteered seemed fearless—and unlike any missionaries I had ever known or imagined. They worked with the youth of Santa Ana, organized peaceful protests, and tried to protect their young parishioners from the government death squads targeting the opposition. I accompanied Father Bill Schmidt and Father John Halbert on home visits and hospital calls and to youth gatherings where I met Salvadorans, most of them younger than I, who were risking their lives to oppose the government. I would walk through the neighborhoods with the priests and talk late into the night about the political struggles of Central America, the devastation they had witnessed, and their conviction that active protests were required for social justice and political change. The Maryknoll priests were committed to justice on a very local level, and they were placing themselves in harm's way to force change. I had grown up as a Catholic but had been drawn to a Protestant church in inner-city Detroit as a medical student because of its strong sense of social mission. To me, a belief in God was a belief in humanity, and it mandated action: free clinics and soup kitchens as social missions just made sense. But later during medical school, I began to question everything about the underpinnings of organized religion. What I saw of liberation theology in El Salvador, however, gave me a new respect for these religious leaders and their impact on their communities. They were driven to action by their faith, and their commitment was impressive. After a month there, I left El Salvador humbled.

I would soon be returning to the nation that was partially responsible for the misery there, though most Americans couldn't even find the country on the map. But for all their dedication and commitment, the Maryknoll priests could not stop the government. As Charlie Clements understood, true change required more than local activism—it also required the mobilization of public opinion and political pressure.

The final stop on my world tour was Geneva, Switzerland, birthplace of the International Committee of the Red Cross (ICRC) and the Geneva Conventions, and the center of the aid world. Geneva hosts the headquarters of many major relief organizations, including the most important UN agencies tackling the humanitarian consequences of war and disaster. Public health emergencies around the world at the time were creating a huge demand for assistance, and relief groups large and small, public and private, were responding. I wanted to know how major agencies like the Office of the UN High Commissioner for Refugees, the Office of the UN Disaster Relief Coordinator, and the World Health Organization planned their responses and coordinated their efforts.

As part of a research project, I developed a survey of major aid agencies and interviewed members of dozens of organizations involved in emergency humanitarian aid. I then conducted a series of structured interviews with the leads of several of the most influential aid agencies to understand the mechanisms they had in place to coordinate their efforts in crisis. I was surprised by what I found. Most of these UN agencies seemed to have little connection with aid workers on the ground and no clear mechanisms for coordinating humanitarian relief with each other. Almost all coordination activity took place in the field and was entirely ad hoc. At the headquarters level, these agencies seemed insular and protectionist rather than open to working together and sharing information and resources. Several UN representatives openly told me that the aid system was broken and that there was a desperate need to create new ways of working collectively among UN leadership.

A year after my visit to Geneva, British journalist Graham Hancock issued a harsh indictment of the growing international aid industry in his book *The Lords of Poverty: The Power, Prestige, and Corruption of the International Aid Business.* Hancock characterized major donors, including the World Bank, the United Nations, the United States Agency for International Development (USAID), and the British Department for International Development as corrupt, secretive, and wholly unaccountable. In the introduction to the book, Hancock quoted Bob Geldof, who, even after the massive success of Live Aid, had grown frustrated with the waste and inefficiency of the West's attempts to provide aid in Africa and called humanitarian aid "a perversion of the act of human generosity."[3] But in 1988, I had no personal context for understanding the ways that the aid community was and wasn't working. I needed a meaningful, practical immersion in the field in order to understand it from the ground up. But further exploration of the aid world would have to wait until after I completed my emergency medicine residency at the University of Illinois at Chicago.

Residency is a concentrated period of intense development for a young physician; a full immersion in clinical medicine. This journey takes a newly graduated medical student and molds him or her into a confident, independent clinician. For the three years of residency, my life was dedicated to keeping up with my training, learning a new specialty, becoming a real doctor, and trying not to kill or injure anyone in the process. My social life all but ceased. Mail piled up at home. And more than once I fell asleep at stoplights while driving home from being on call overnight.

Emergency medicine residents start out by rotating through major specialties like surgery, obstetrics, pediatrics, and internal medicine before settling into specific training within the emergency departments, where decisions to act or not act have very real human consequences. As interns begin to advance, they experience the terror of not knowing and the thrill of learning on the spot. They manage patients under the watchful presence of senior residents and attending physicians, slowly developing both competence and confidence. As residents progress through their second year, they expand their base of knowledge, experience, and skill. These young doctors hopefully develop confidence, but not arrogance. Much of emergency medicine training aims to develop thoughtful physicians who have the self assurance to act decisively and the humility to never stop learning. For me, residency was a period of intense and gratifying intellectual and emotional growth, even if I had little time for anything else. Chicago's ERs were like those of Detroit: big and busy, with a constant stream of ambulances, patients, and drama. Days at the hospital would begin at 6:00 a.m. and finish at 7:00 or 8:00 p.m. On-call days would mean all-nighters every third or fourth night, admitting patients and managing emergencies on the floor. Rotations in the ER were ten or twelve hours of constant movement, with entire shifts going by without a chance to eat or go to the bathroom.

Although I couldn't see it at the time, my emergency medicine residency was preparing me for a future career in humanitarian medicine, a field that, like emergency medicine, was still new. I was learning to deal with all kinds of personalities and egos, and how to manage them in order to help my patients. I learned to work harder and longer than I ever thought I could, and to stay focused despite exhaustion. I learned to be a fierce and persistent advocate for my patients, and to honor and respect the nurses, technicians, and other members of my team. Finally, I learned to stay flexible, positive, and confident in the face of adversity. Despite these valuable lessons, though, applying them to the humanitarian field would have to wait. There was no escaping residency.

There was also no escaping life. I met my future wife on my first on-call night as an intern at Illinois Masonic Hospital. Julie Arnold, a graduate of Northwestern University's Medill School of Journalism, was exploring her interest in medicine by working as a clerk in the emergency room at Illinois Masonic. Over the course of her year there, she realized that she wanted to trade her keyboard for a scalpel, and so she applied to medical school at the University of Illinois at Chicago.

That first night on call at Masonic, I went down to the ER to attend a trauma patient, a young man with a stab wound to the abdomen. As an intern, most of my work was "scut," the most undesirable jobs performed by the most junior member of the team. As I ran around gathering blood bank forms for an operation, one of the physicians told me to ask the clerk for a particular form. I walked around a corner and nearly ran into Julie, who was staffing the registration desk. I looked at her, stammered, forgot what I came for, and left without saying a word. The attending physician saw the look on my face and laughed out loud. I spent the rest of the evening finding excuses to go back down to the ER, trying to find out that clerk's name and number. Returning home the following evening after an exhausting all-night call, I told my roommate that I had found the woman I was going to marry. Then I collapsed into bed.

Julie and I saw each other only sporadically during my internship, but we dated more steadily after she started medical school the following year and we soon fell in love. I knew I had found a partner in both life and medicine. Julie was and is smart, beautiful, funny, and opinionated. She had a way of challenging me and encouraging me at the same time. She also seemed to accept my vague notions of working abroad. We spent long nights talking about our shared sense of mission and the duty to go out into the world to effect change. She became my sounding board for every seemingly silly idea and encouraged me to make them happen. The two easiest decisions in my early life were choosing emergency medicine as a specialty and choosing Julie as my partner.

Julie and I spent hours talking about where our combined careers would take us. Every week, we would walk to D'Agostino's, a little Italian restaurant near our Wrigleyville apartment. We'd sit together on one side of a booth, looking at a world atlas and planning our future travels. I'm sure I looked like a considerable travel geek as I traced my fingers along the borders of the same African countries I had dreamed about in that Michigan hospital cafeteria two decades before during my mother's illness. But not only did Julie humor me; she joined in the scheming. We decided that after I finished residency and worked for a year to save enough to cover our school debts, she would take a leave from medical school, and we would sell or store everything and spend a year abroad exploring the field of global health.

As I looked for opportunities overseas, I reflected on the reasons I had chosen the field of emergency medicine: the complex nature of emergencies, the sense of contributing to the growth of a new medical specialty, and the challenge of coordinating diverse services to care for patients. I searched for work that would help me explore the field. My introduction to disaster relief in India, to conflict in El Salvador, and to the UN agencies in Geneva had given me a brief glimpse into the massive complex of international aid, but I wanted a deeper dive into the field.

Before I finished my residency, events unfolded in the Middle East that would eventually change the aid community in profound ways. In August 1990, Iraqi forces invaded the small neighboring state of Kuwait. Five months later, US and allied troops launched Operation Desert Storm to push the Iraqis out of Kuwait. That objective was accomplished and a ceasefire declared within six weeks. But as coalition troops withdrew in March 1991, the Kurdish rebellion—which was encouraged by the CIA and expected to receive US support—took up arms against Saddam Hussein's regime. Tens of thousands were killed before Hussein crushed the monthlong uprising. More than a million Kurds fled north toward Turkey and Iran. Ultimately, nearly 500,000 refugees were trapped in harsh mountain terrain, prompting a large-scale humanitarian mission to protect them. On April 5, 1991, the United Nations passed Resolution 688, condemning the Iraqi repression of the Kurds and insisting that Iraq allow international humanitarian aid into the Kurdistan region. The aid effort, led by the United Kingdom, the United States, and France, was dubbed Operation Provide Comfort. The joint military–civilian effort protected Kurds from Iraqi governmental forces and allowed them to return to their homes under a no-fly zone. The effort was a clear success. It also led to a bold move by the UN General Assembly in December 1991 to adopt Resolution 46/182, establishing the United Nations Office for the Coordination of Humanitarian Affairs (OCHA). This resolution also led to the creation of the Inter-Agency Standing Committee (IASC), a UN-led organization that aimed to facilitate coordination, funding, and policy in humanitarian action.

Humanitarian crises like the Ethiopian famine and the Kurdish refugee crisis were increasingly recognized as acute, massive public health emergencies. Epidemiologists Michael J. Toole and Ronald J. Waldman of the US Centers for Disease Control and Prevention (CDC) developed the concept that when mortality rates rise to twice the baseline rate for a particular population, a humanitarian emergency exists—war and natural disasters create conditions where people are displaced, property destroyed, and access to food and health services is disrupted. In these settings, death rates skyrocket, especially among the very young and very old, and extraordinary international relief efforts should be deployed. I knew there was no real comparison between the ghettos of Detroit and Chicago and the refugee camps of Sudan, but my emergency medicine experience suggested a common thread: poverty, instability, and political impotence left people more vulnerable to violence.

As humanitarians learned how to respond to large-scale emergencies, they expanded their scope of activity beyond the provision of food, shelter, and health care. It has been increasingly recognized that emergency assistance alone can't make a community or country whole again. Short-term aid cannot stabilize a nation and set it on the road toward recovery. Wars and natural disasters create vicious cycles of political and economic instability that can impede economic development for decades. Of the forty nations at the bottom of the UN's Human Development Index—a statistical measure of life expectancy, education, income, and other factors—65 percent have experienced recurrent war and disaster, leading to perpetual underdevelopment, poverty, and political turmoil.

As aid changed and evolved, so did the perception of aid workers. In the 1980s, relief workers from Western nations had been seen as heroes riding to the rescue, but during the 1990s, their roles became more complicated and attracted more criticism. In the wake of the Cold War, several new intrastate conflicts erupted. Western nations increasingly used humanitarian aid as a diplomatic tool and a replacement for political or military intervention—a heavy weight for those in the field to bear. Suddenly international NGOs were asked to step forward to provide emergency aid in highly volatile settings where there was no political will to act militarily.

As the UN adapted its mission to include the growing number of refugees and displaced populations around the world, many of its agencies began partnering with NGOs. This set off a period of explosive growth in the number of NGOs. At the UN's founding in 1945, there were 2,865 known groups categorized as NGOs; by 1990, that number had nearly quintupled to 13,591. By the late 1990s, nearly $8 billion per year in donations was being pumped into the aid industry. Aid was in vogue, and NGOs were seen as the all-purpose vehicle not only for humanitarian relief, but also for human rights, peace building, and disarmament. Aid workers were celebrated as global do-gooders and moved deeper than ever before into conflict zones to deliver aid and negotiate on behalf of civilians in conflict.

But even as aid flexed its muscles in Kurdistan and elsewhere, the limits of emergency humanitarian relief were becoming clear. The infusion into conflict zones of humanitarian relief alone could create neither stability nor an adequate foundation for economic recovery, and aid was also exploited. The next decade would see humanitarian aid systematically manipulated by combatants to gain protection, food, resources, and weapons, and increasingly aid would be abused to prolong conflicts and gain public influence. Providing emergency humanitarian assistance was not as simple as making airdrops or food deliveries. As part of a larger ecosystem of power, politics, economics, and development strategy, it could not be seen in isolation from a political solution.

Julie and I departed in 1992 for our yearlong exploration of global health. We did research in the United Kingdom and medical informatics in Russia, and ultimately ended up in Tenwek Hospital, a mission hospital in rural Kenya. Near the end of a month there, I was asked to join a medical relief team organized by Samaritan's Purse, a North Carolina–based NGO. The organization was relatively new to field operations, and it was establishing a new program in Somalia, where the political environment was highly charged and quite unpredictable. The relief team was headed to Mogadishu, the Somali capital, a daunting testing ground. While many aid agencies were active in and around Mogadishu, the security situation was constantly changing. The medical and public health needs of the communities outside of the capital were profound, and access to those most affected was often restricted. I had little firsthand knowledge of the situation on the ground, yet as I walked onto the tarmac of the airport to board the C-130 cargo plane, I had no hesitation, just excitement. I suddenly felt different, as if I were stepping off a precipice into a brand new world and new phase of my life.

In January 1991, a coalition of armed opposition forces overthrew the twenty-two-year military dictatorship of Somali president Mohamed Siad Barre, and the country sank into a ferocious civil war. As rival clans battled for power, tens of thousands were killed, and the agricultural economy was devastated. Once again, war led to famine, and starvation and malnutrition swept the country. International aid groups began moving thousands of tons of food through the port city of Mogadishu. Clans swept in to extort the food aid, selling goods for weapons. The food shipments were fueling the war and the famine.

By 1992, more than 300,000 Somalis had died and 1.5 million faced starvation. Nearly five million people, more than half the population of Somalia, were completely dependent on food aid. Increased international attention prompted many aid groups to set up operations in the country. In August 1992, President George H. W. Bush announced Operation Provide Relief to secure aid delivery to Somalia. The UN-sanctioned effort employed American military personnel to transport and distribute relief shipments. These efforts proved inadequate. Increasing clan warfare and the growing aggressiveness of armed groups undermined attempts to secure food delivery, and food aid continued to fuel the conflict. In December 1992 Provide Relief gave way to Operation Restore Hope, with US soldiers deployed to provide security and ensure that aid reached starving Somalis. The images of suffering beamed out of Somalia by news cameras created public pressure to act. A growing number of organizations entered the country, as did multinational military forces, to work in the complex and dangerous climate of the clan-divided nation.

As I departed Nairobi en route to Mogadishu, I met Kenney Isaacs from Samaritan's Purse, who briefed me on the planned medical response in Somalia. Ken is a dedicated Christian and a deeply experienced relief expert with an unusual combination of common sense and courage. He had originally worked as a well driller but proved to be a remarkably creative and persistent leader with a natural ability to negotiate access to some of the most challenging environments. He was largely responsible for building the international relief program at Samaritan's Purse. He was later appointed director of the Office of Foreign Disaster Assistance (OFDA), the US government's primary humanitarian relief agency. Over the next twenty years, I would work with and learn from Ken. Through our work in conflict areas around the world, he would emerge as one of my best friends and most important mentors.

His invitation to lead a team to Somalia was the realization of my childhood aspiration of being a doctor in Africa. But there were many times over the next six months that it felt more like a mistake. My career has since taken me to war zones in the Balkans, Rwanda, Sudan, Congo, North Korea and Iraq, but Mogadishu remains the most hostile place I've ever worked.

* * *

THE MOMENT THE BACK HATCH of the C-130 cargo opened at the militarized airport in Mogadishu, a wave of intense heat hit me. The hot wind blew fine red dust that covered me before I even reached the tarmac. I knew this place would be unlike any other I had been to before. UNOSOM, the United Nations Operation in Somalia, controlled the airport, and the property was surrounded by military vehicles, sandbagged posts, and razor wire. It was a hive of NGO and UN activity, with shipments of relief goods and aid workers arriving hourly. I hitched a ride with the Save the Children convoy and stayed in their walled compound until I could find my way to our headquarters. The rest of the team, including Julie, arrived the next day, and I joined them at the Samaritan's Purse compound. During our first night there, we heard yelling and running and machine gunfire just outside of our room. After the first crackles of gunfire, I realized that all the windows to the bedroom were open. I yelled to Julie to roll off the bed and lie flat on the floor. Keeping the lights off, we crawled on our hands and knees out of the room and up the building's two flights of stairs to avoid being shot through the open windows along the stairway. The gunshots now sounded like they were all around the house. We scrambled our way onto the flat roof, where we found the other members of our team. A moment later, one of the surgeons appeared carrying an AK-47, and we all reflexively ducked as he swung up the stairs. I wondered which was more dangerous, the shooting down below or the gun-wielding surgeon on the roof. He laid the gun down, and we called the UN compound to report the event. By then, the gunfire seemed to have stopped, but we all waited for what seemed like hours before returning to bed.

I struggle to write about Somalia in ways that are not cliché. As my first humanitarian mission, it was so incredibly different and larger than life. The ruined city of Mogadishu had a hellish feeling, starting with its temperatures, which reached 110 degrees Fahrenheit. The buildings were pockmarked with holes from bullets and rocket-propelled grenades (RPGs). Somali militiamen wearing sunglasses and toting the universal AK-47s patrolled the streets in "Technicals"—Toyota pickup trucks that had been modified by welding large-caliber machine guns onto their beds. Even the peaceful-looking waters of the Indian Ocean teemed with sharks. One day, Abdulahi, the Somali manager of all of the compound's staff, told me that we needed to have more weapons, even though we had hired security guards to protect the compound. "Go to Bakara and buy some more weapons," he said, "and then show your own guards that you have them." So we went with our security guards to the Bakara Market in central Mogadishu, the largest of the central markets. Bakara was a congested bazaar filled with fruit, trinkets, blankets, hanging meat that was collecting flies, and khat, a locally grown stimulant that looks like cilantro but acts like an amphetamine.

The arms market was surreal. We wove through its crowded, sweltering alleys and were directed to a dark plywood stall that looked like an arsenal. Automatic weapons hung on the walls like groceries. The Kalashnikov rifles, hand grenades, and rocket-propelled grenades were all leftovers from the Soviet era, when weapons had flooded into the country. At one time, it was estimated that there were 300,000 automatic weapons in Mogadishu, about one for every three people in the city.[4] We bought one AK-47 and ammunition for about $250. Over the following weeks, in addition to our medical work, we all took lessons in cleaning, storing, and shooting AK-47s with the US Marines stationed in Somalia. I must admit, however, that it was no comfort to me or any of the staff to have weapons in our home, but they were everywhere in Somalia—a strange reality. About a month later, the weapons shops at the Bakara Market were shut down by UNOSOM forces in an attempt to disarm the citizens of Mogadishu. This ultimately proved to be futile.

As part of the medical team, I helped organize mobile clinics—trucks loaded with medical equipment, supplies, and personnel—that would take us around the capital and to inland towns like Baidoa and Baardheere and their surrounding villages. I also helped select appropriate sites for our clinics and negotiated safe passage with the local elders and warlords. On one memorable day in March 1993, we set up a clinic inside an abandoned movie theater. It was a odd sight. The hot, cavernous old building had its own war wounds—its ceiling was crumbling, the old screen was in tatters, and RPGs had left car-sized holes in its walls—but it was the best available space for our work. My colleagues and I had unpacked and were beginning to set up a station to triage the ill and injured Somalis who had gathered when the leader of one of the warring clans barged in with family members in tow, demanding that we take care of them immediately. We told him, through a translator, that we had to treat the sickest people first, and that his relatives—who seemed comparatively healthy—would have to wait.

Infuriated, the clan leader left. He soon returned with a half-dozen raggedly dressed militiamen carrying AK-47s and chewing khat. Shouting in Somali, the jumpy young men circled around us, rummaged through our supplies, and terrified our patients. When we heard the crack of gunfire outside, I fully expected them to start shooting in the theater. We stopped our triage, and I asked the clan leader to speak privately. After some conversation, we finally agreed that I would treat his wife first. Guards stood by while I quickly examined and treated her with Tylenol for her chronic back pain. I reassured the clan leader that his wife was in good health, and we were allowed to proceed with our clinic. It was the first of many compromises I would have to make in the field for the sake of keeping our relief programs running.

I spent the next several months traveling between Chicago, Nairobi (the base of operation for many international NGOs), and Mogadishu. I had just returned to the United States from Somalia when the infamous "Black Hawk Down" incident occurred, marking the beginning of the end of US military involvement in Somalia. At this time, Mogadishu's most powerful warlord, General Mohamed Farrah Aidid, had denounced the growing foreign presence and shown defiance toward UNOSOM attempts to disarm the clans. Attacks on UN personnel and military escorts had been escalating. On October 3, 1993, the

United States military captured two of Aidid's top lieutenants in an assault in Mogadishu. In the sixteen-hour clash that followed, two Black Hawk helicopters were shot down with RPGs near the notorious Bakara Market. Eighteen US servicemen were killed, and triumphant Somalis dragged the bodies of some American casualties through the streets. The Somali death toll was much higher—1,000 to 1,500, including civilians, by some estimates. The battle would shift public attention away from supporting the relief effort in Somalia, and this shift would influence future aid decisions—most notably in Rwanda.

In this conflict, and in many of the "new wars" of the 1990s, malnutrition and infectious diseases, not bullets and RPGs, were the biggest killers. War and famine had also fractured the Somali family structure. Most of the country's husbands and fathers were away fighting or dead, while the women remained behind with small children. In the face of growing insecurity and persistent famine, hundreds of thousands sought refuge at food distribution sites around the cities, where makeshift camps sprang up. At one camp in Mogadishu, several thousand refugees cobbled together shelters from plastic sheeting, canvas bags, and bits of string and wire. It was there that I met a Somali woman who would change the way I viewed my humanitarian work and who gave me the most valuable lesson of my humanitarian career.

Our team was conducting a formal health and nutrition survey in the displacement camp, screening children between one and five years old for malnutrition, though we could see at a glance that most were underfed and covered with sores from scabies. We had created two work stations shaded by tarps and had the mothers line up with their children so we could measure the child's middle upper-arm circumference with a colored tape, a way of determining whether he or she suffered from mild, moderate, or severe wasting due to malnutrition. Then we took the children to a bathing area, stood them in a series of tubs, scrubbed them, and treated them for scabies. Finally, we gave the mothers medication to prevent the roundworms and tapeworms that were endemic in the camp.

We worked our way through hundreds of children, measuring, categorizing, and noting who required supplemental feeding. As we were moving the children through the treatment stations, a girl came forward in significantly worse condition than the others. Her name was Fatima, and her bloated belly and stunted size indicated that she suffered from kwashiorkor, a severe type of malnutrition caused by profound protein deficiency. She told our interpreter that she was around five years old, but she looked like a toddler. She was covered with flies that clumped on abscesses from scabies, and her hair was reddish and brittle from vitamin deficiency. She clearly needed intensive therapeutic feeding in a specialized center in order to survive, and so we called a vehicle, planning to bring her to the ICRC therapeutic feeding center.

Through an interpreter, I asked to speak to the child's mother. None of the women standing by responded. I asked again, but received no response. Finally, someone in the crowd told the translator that Fatima had no mother; she was an orphan.

"Who takes care of her?" I asked. The women shrugged.

"No one," a voice replied.

Irritated at their seeming indifference, I persisted: "Someone must be helping this child."

After an uncomfortable silence, one of the women motioned to me to come with her. She grabbed me firmly by the shirtsleeve and pulled me along, saying nothing as we wove between the rough plastic shelters until we arrived at hers. She opened the flap, stared at me hard, and briskly gestured for me to look inside. I bent down to peer into the six-by-six-foot enclosure of plastic and burlap, and saw a small bag of rice, a cooking pot, and three small children sitting on the dirt floor. One of them was coughing. When I stood back up, the woman fixed her gaze on me again and turned both of her palms to the sky in a gesture of helplessness.

Finally, I understood. I knew nothing of her struggles. I had come from relative wealth and privilege, had never known hunger or feared for my life. I carried a passport in my back pocket and could leave at any time. I had been indignant at the indifference of these women, but they were faced with an impossible dilemma: they sought to keep their own children alive and had no way of helping as another's child starved in their midst. It was a terrible decision they were forced to make, and I was immediately ashamed of my naïveté, suddenly and painfully aware that despite my sincere desire to help, I had come woefully unprepared. I realized that despite my training, I was ill-equipped to understand the conditions here.

And I wasn't alone. I realized that most of us, despite our past experiences and good intentions, had little idea of the complexities we were facing in Somalia. Even the most experienced organizations were not ready to tackle the compounding threats of severe malnutrition, war trauma, and infectious disease all at once in the most challenging environment imaginable.

My experiences in Somalia led to an epiphany about my future. I began thinking seriously about the systemic changes needed to better prepare aid workers and strengthen international humanitarian response. The civilians caught in this and other conflicts deserved better.

The suffering of a malnourished refugee in the squalor of a camp is an affront to human dignity. That dignity is something we all possess and must fight to preserve. Perhaps now I also could better understand my patients in inner-city Detroit or Chicago, where the oppression of poverty and culture of violence drives them to helplessness. The struggle to promote human dignity was not only to be fought in Somalia, but also closer to home.

3

CAREER
HUMANITARIAN

SOMALIA WAS A PIVOTAL MOMENT IN MY CAREER. IT was also a turning point for humanitarian intervention in general. The military–civilian humanitarian experiment had failed. Aid was no longer simply aid; it was a political and diplomatic tool, whether practitioners liked it or not, and it wasn't working. The rules that had once applied to international humanitarian organizations in the field seemed to be unraveling. Unarmed aid workers were no longer seen as neutral, but were viewed as part of the Western "occupation" of Somalia. NGO compounds and convoys increasingly came under attack. Aid workers were threatened and obstructed, and there was no longer a safe way to operate in the country.

My experiences in Somalia were also humbling. I saw that I lacked any real understanding of the complex political and security implications of aid. I had been wholly unprepared for the challenges of medical work within the health system of a failed state and an unstable environment. After Somalia, I became convinced that to improve humanitarian aid as an industry, we needed to teach leaders and practitioners how to understand their environment and make better decisions. We needed to invest in professional education. Aid was still crucial, but its current framework also seemed deeply flawed. The aid community was learning and evolving though its involvement in complex environments like Somalia, and so was I. It was clear that I needed more experience. The next opportunity to grow as a humanitarian would soon present itself.

The impending collapse of the Soviet Union in the late 1980s was evident in the Russian retreat from Afghanistan and the fall of the Berlin Wall in 1989. By the end of 1991, the USSR had disintegrated. It was a hopeful time for democratic movements. For the humanitarian aid world, the retraction of Soviet interests meant greater access to areas that had previously been off-limits. The United Nations began to play a more active role in diplomacy, and UN military operations soon became the answer to resolving small conflicts and clearing the way for the civilian humanitarian aid community to make a significant impact.

That hopefulness was short-lived. The end of the Cold War closed the curtain on a number of East–West proxy conflicts, but "new wars" quickly took the global stage. These were civil conflicts marked by rebel militias, assaults on civilians, and ethnic discrimination. Conflicts throughout the Horn of Africa, West Africa, Eastern Europe, and the Middle East grew in complexity and ferocity. By 1993, there were officially forty-seven active armed conflicts around the world, in places like Somalia, Sudan, and the former Yugoslavia; forty-three of them were civil wars. The humanitarian consequences of these conflicts, including civilian casualties, ethnic cleansing, and genocide, became known in the aid world as "complex humanitarian emergencies." The suffering they created was immense, and access to threatened populations was hindered by the occupation of civilian territories by militias who sought to control and manipulate the flow of aid resources.

This was a time of explosive growth of humanitarian aid agencies and UN interventions. Instead of calling for an expansion of international military presence in these new conflicts, Western governments increased the budgets of many aid agencies. Funding for humanitarian relief increased steadily in the 1990s, although the percentage of the overall US budget spent on aid declined to the lowest level in decades.[1] New aid organizations appeared, such as the International Medical Corps, and existing aid agencies like Save the Children, Oxfam, and Médecins Sans Frontières grew. The expansion of international aid as a replacement for political or military solutions came to be known as the "humanitarian fig leaf," a euphemism for the use of aid as an (inadequate) substitute for meaningful political or military action by the West. Aid agencies could deliver food, medicine, and relief supplies, but could never solve the core problems that made these basic resources so scarce.

The crisis-packed 1990s sparked a transformation in the growing aid community. The UN Security Council stepped up its interventions to protect threatened civilians, even without the consent of the governments in a given conflict zone. The United Nations also rapidly expanded its function as a global police force. From 1945, when the

United Nations was established, to 1988, only five peacekeeping missions were authorized. In the five years from 1989 to 1994, the United Nations undertook twenty new peacekeeping missions. In addition, the United Nations increased its ability to manage and fund relief efforts, creating important committees for coordinating aid and passing a series of measures to better finance humanitarian action.

The 1990s were also a turning point for civilian aid agencies. The 1991 combined military–civilian relief effort in Kurdistan ushered in a new era of cooperation in humanitarian efforts. The ghastly famine in Somalia, and the struggles of both civilian and military missions there, completely changed political and public attitudes toward international humanitarian interventions. Eventually, the loss of eighteen soldiers in the 1993 Battle of Mogadishu turned public sentiment against military humanitarian intervention.

As I gained experience in the field, I learned to respect the complexity of emergency aid. Each conflict or disaster was unique, but there were emerging common themes that could be used for planning and improving responses. The challenges I faced as a physician in a war zone brought me face-to-face with some of the most pivotal issues in the humanitarian world. For instance, from the sterile safety of a classroom or on the pages of a textbook, the idea of international law in war and conflict and the protocols of the Geneva Conventions are theoretical abstractions. But in the field, they take on very tangible and practical importance. My experiences in Somalia, for example, showed me that protecting human rights and ensuring access to civilians are very local and practical aims, and must be at the heart of what aid agencies do. The civilian aid community must advocate—from the front lines—for civilians caught in conflict. In reality, this is quite difficult.

The limitations of our ability to protect and provide for civilians became painfully evident to me during the Yugoslavia conflict, when Serbian- and Croatian-led campaigns of "ethnic cleansing" against the Bosnians were all too reminiscent of the world's failure to protect civilians from the Nazi-era practices that had impacted my father so profoundly.

The country of Yugoslavia was born in the aftermath of World War I, folding together a host of ethnic, cultural, religious, and national identities into a fragile union. Yugoslavia was composed of six major regions, the largest of which was Serbia, in the east. Serbia controlled most of the nation's military assets, and Serbian nationalists occupied other areas of the country. Bosnia-Herzegovina, located geographically in the center of the country, was a complex patchwork of Croatians, Bosnian Muslims, and Serbs. Yugoslavia survived the tumult of World War II and the rise of the Iron Curtain thanks to the iron-handed dictatorship of Josip Tito. After Tito died in 1980, the tension between the various parts of Yugoslavia began to rise. In 1991, when the Soviet Union collapsed, so did Yugoslavia.

Croatia and Slovenia, the westernmost regions in Yugoslavia, declared themselves independent nations in 1991. When Bosnia-Herzegovina followed suit, Serbian forces attacked to secure Serb territory within Bosnia. The conflict escalated into a multi-directional civil war that involved three major groups: Serbs, Croatians, and Bosnian Muslims, known as Bosniaks. Lasting for ten years, it was the most deadly conflict in Europe since the end of World War II, killing over 120,000 people, mostly civilians, and displacing over 2.2 million. Civilians fleeing Srebrenica and other war zones became, in the parlance of the aid community, "internally displaced people," trapped inside Yugoslavia, refugees within their own country. The Yugoslav War was a macabre carnival of human rights abuses and atrocities. The international community struggled to effectively unify against bold Serbian aggression, which included the rape of an estimated 20,000 to 50,000 women, mass murder of civilians, and Nazi-style concentration camps.

One particularly gruesome act of genocide occurred in Srebrenica, a city in eastern Bosnia-Herzegovina. In April 1993, the majority-Muslim enclave of Srebrenica was declared a "safe area" by the United Nations and placed under the protection of Dutch UN peacekeepers. The population of the region had become swollen with refugees seeking the protection of the United Nations. In 1995, Serbian forces under the command of Ratko Mladić attacked Srebrenica, defying the UN safe area decree. The battalion of Dutch peacekeepers was unable to stop the advancing Serbian troops and called for NATO air support to deter the Serbian advance. When no support was realized, Mladić and his troops marched into Srebrenica, isolated the civilian men, and systematically executed them. Serbian troops continued on a spree of attacks, pulling women and girls out of the group of refugees in a campaign of mass rape. Over 8,000 Bosnians were killed, and 30,000 more were expelled from the city. The Srebrenica massacre led to countless reports of war crimes and, eventually, indictments. It was the worst atrocity on European soil since World War II.

Probably the most high-profile example of Serbian aggression was the siege of Sarajevo, the capital of Bosnia-Herzegovina, for nearly four years, from 1992 to 1996. It was the longest siege in modern history, three times longer than the siege of Stalingrad. Nearly 12,000 well-armed Serbian fighters surrounded the city and terrorized the population with artillery, mortars, rocket launchers, heavy machine guns, and long-range sniper rifles. With access to the city blocked and no diplomatic solution in sight, civilians starved, froze, and remained trapped in their homes for fear of exposing themselves to sniper fire. They burned furniture and strips of wooden floors to heat their homes, and had to depend on corridors of foreign aid to prevent starvation.

Aid agencies' access to the city was tenuous. The UN flight service in and out of Sarajevo, where I traveled in 1993 to work at the city's State Hospital, was known as "Maybe Airlines," a tongue-in-cheek reference to the unreliability of flights into the city. I found transport within the city to be even more difficult to navigate. It was dangerous to move anywhere outside. Mortars were routinely lobbed into central neighborhoods, and the streets were lined with forty-foot shipping containers placed end-to-end to provide a barrier behind which the citizens of Sarajevo could venture out to get food or collect water. The UN Protection Forces (UNPROFOR) worked to create a complex web of passages for humanitarian access into Sarajevo and other major cities besieged by war. As in most conflicts, restricted access meant restrictions in health care, and medical services in enclaves like Sarajevo suffered.

In the winter of 1993, I worked as an emergency physician in a war hospital in a town called Nova Bila in central Bosnia. The facility was an improvised hospital in the Fra. Mato Nikolić Franciscan church, also called the Nova Bila Hospital for War Wounded. The facility was in Travnik, a Croat-held enclave with a total population of about 60,000 people. The Travnik area was completely encircled by Bosniak forces. Roads and access points were blocked or mined, and supplies were severely restricted. Most of the physicians and medical personnel in the region had been forced to flee, leaving the makeshift hospital desperately understaffed. The hospital was close to the front line of conflict, and it was shelled and shot at frequently. To protect the patients and medical staff inside, the outside of the hospital was covered with twenty-foot planks on all sides to prevent snipers from shooting doctors and patients and to keep shrapnel from mortar blasts from blowing through the windows.

By the time I arrived, the hospital was under severe strain. The Croatian physicians were effectively isolated, with no ability to leave the hospital or obtain supplies or relief. The main ward was the church sanctuary, which was freezing cold and lit mainly by rows of stained-glass windows behind the planks. The operating theaters were concrete block rooms in the basement. Nova Bila was a punishing environment for patients and staff. To keep the generators running for surgeries, fuel was severely restricted, which meant no heat. The surgeons worked long, cold hours with cracked and bleeding hands. Food for the patients and staff was rationed. Every normal resource, from bandages to blankets, was extremely limited. Every member of the medical staff was malnourished and suffered greatly through the long Eastern European winter. The patients in the hospital fared no better: with no heat and limited food, it was a harsh environment for recovery.

I arrived at the hospital in a UN armored personnel carrier after crossing several checkpoints. The Norwegian convoy that transported me required everyone to wear full flak jackets and white helmets. After arriving at the hospital compound, I changed into scrubs and met the medical staff in the living room of the former rectory. They talked about several recent battles very close to the hospital, as well as the strain on fuel, supplies, and medication. I had brought with me two trunks of sutures, surgical equipment, and dressing supplies. It was a drop in the bucket, considering their needs, but they were nevertheless grateful and gracious. The lead physician, Dr. Branimir Kuliš, welcomed me to their staff. A senior surgeon who looked gaunt from the long months of work but had an air of both determination and kindness, he appeared to be a quiet, thoughtful man who commanded the respect of the medical team. We sat hunched over an old coffee table with the rest of the medical staff and drank Turkish coffee, smoked cigarettes, and took a welcoming shot of slivovitz, the ubiquitous (and horrible) plum brandy found all over Eastern Europe.

As if timed to our toast, a mortar round hit close to the hospital. Several more explosions boomed nearby on the front line of the conflict. The surgeons looked at each other, exhausted, and stood up to prepare for another volley of patients. Just as we stood up, a reporter and a cameraman from CNN came into the hospital. They had somehow heard there was an American doctor working there and smelled a story. At first I declined. I had only just arrived and had not even begun to work.

But the hospital director and the staff felt that international coverage could generate support for the hospital, and so I acquiesced, and the journalists followed me into the operating room, where I assisted the surgical staff in several operations. After seven hours in the OR, we walked out into the cold hospital to conduct rounds on patients in the dark: checking wounds, managing medications, listening to stories. The evening dinner was bread and soup, and I was famished. Still, I felt guilty for eating when food was so scarce. I finally went to my tiny, dark, unheated room, placed my flak jacket in the window in case a mortar round exploded close by, and shut my eyes on the end of my first day in Nova Bila. I was excited to be there, but lying on my cot in the cold, I wondered how I could really be helpful in this struggle. I was a young, foreign doctor in the middle of a war zone, trying to help create a safe place for people whose struggles I could not begin to imagine.

Running a hospital for casualties at Nova Bila was hard enough. But we also had to serve a large civilian population with no other access to health care. The hospital staff did treat those who had suffered from trauma, but most of the patients were there for pneumonia, heart attacks, and routine surgical care. Nova Bila took all comers, including war wounded. One morning while I was working, a major battle took place nearby. The hospital was rocked by mortar fire, and soon after, around thirty Croatian soldiers delivered a dozen injured patients to the hospital. Armed, uniformed soldiers entered the halls of the hospital, the emergency ward, and the grounds, turning a civilian medical facility into a military war hospital. The medical staff quickly met to discuss how to handle this large influx of patients, and especially the arrival of Croatian soldiers straight from the battlefield, which was a very real threat to the hospital's claim of neutrality. If Nova Bila was perceived as militarized, it would become a greater target for Bosniak fighters. The soldiers also acted as an intimidating presence for the medical staff and patients, and they showed no signs of leaving.

After a quick huddle, Dr. Perić, another lead surgeon, met with the military commander and negotiated a solution. We would, of course, accept and treat all wounded patients, but we needed to "demilitarize" the hospital. Injured soldiers would be changed out of their military uniforms and into civilian attire. The Croatian soldiers agreed to leave the hospital grounds. After seeing the soldiers out, we continued to operate into the night by the light of the generators.

Despite extreme shortages of fuel, food, medical supplies, and personnel, the hospital achieved remarkable success in dealing with devastating trauma. During the Yugoslav War, the risk of sustaining a critical penetrating injury from direct gunshot wound was nearly three times that of Vietnam, with higher rates of head injury. This led to death rates higher than those seen in Vietnam hospitals, comparable to rates at war hospitals in Lebanon and Afghanistan. Furthermore, despite the flood of war wounded, the hospital's leadership achieved a small miracle in keeping Nova Bila neutral—which meant fewer direct attacks on the facility itself and a safer environment for civilians.

My experience in Bosnia taught me several new lessons about my place in the aid field. After days of travel, and the danger of passing though lines of conflict, I felt that my work in the hospital was only marginally useful to my Croatian medical colleagues, hampered as I was by language and cultural barriers and a lack of familiar tools. Directly working as a physician may have been useful, but there were likely better ways to make an impact. I also felt that my presence and my support of those heroic local physicians were the more important contributions. My presence in Nova Bila brought attention to their struggle and assured them that they were not alone, and any support I could give to the local doctors, nurses, technicians, and staff who had dedicated themselves to helping people in the most challenging of circumstances was well worth the investment. Reflecting on my various missions in Nova Bila and Sarajevo, I was once again confronted with the question of what the best approach was to help the most: direct service, teaching, or some greater policy effort. I returned home with a new respect for my medical colleagues in the field, and a renewed commitment to do better.

Coming home after several intense weeks in the field made for a disorienting contrast. Work in the field was all-consuming, and it was sometimes quite difficult to resume normal life. I tried to pick up where I had left off, diving back into family life without any downtime. It was not always a smooth transition. I remember the frustration of being stuck in Sarajevo, awaiting a flight on "Maybe Airlines," desperate to get home for Julie's medical school graduation. As was common in UN flights, I was bumped off the manifest by UN staff who took priority, and I missed the graduation, arriving home two days later. I know she was disappointed, yet, like so many other times when I had been working abroad with little or no contact, she was remarkably supportive. She always struck a wonderful balance of being patient with long stretches apart and still being anxious for my return. Especially in these early days of long travel and virtual silence from the field, Julie really understood that this work was more than just time away; it was an exploration of what I hoped to become. I depended on her for much more than moral support; she allowed me to walk back into the arms of normalcy after some very strange and unsettling events that would have otherwise taken a heavy psychological toll. Having worked in the field herself, she understood its challenges, both logistical and emotional, and remained my home base.

As difficult as it was to move between two worlds, the growing portfolio of field experience I was gaining was extremely valuable and transformed my academic medical practice. I was a better, more thoughtful doctor and came to appreciate the value of providing care to individual patients. My fieldwork also drove me to integrate what I did in the field with my research and teaching at home, and to combine the two halves of my professional life into the academic pursuit of humanitarian science. This blending allowed me to use the field as a laboratory. I started asking key, as-yet-unanswered questions about the provision of humanitarian medicine. What are the most efficient ways of setting up emergency health services for refugees? Are there best practices in reestablishing health systems? How can doctors and nurses most effectively work in conflict settings? This combination also expanded my own understanding of the complicated environment that aid workers face. The rigors of my medical education and training as an emergency physician told me that the aid world needed a more rigorous and evidence-based approach to humanitarian aid. In a matter of months, events unfolding in the Great Lakes region of Africa would show just how urgent this need was.

4

GROWING CHALLENGES

THE 1994 RWANDAN GENOCIDE EMERGED FROM A civil war fought between the Hutu-led government and the Tutsi-led Rwandan Patriotic Front (RPF). Ethnic tensions in Rwanda had been building for several decades, with their roots in the Belgian colonial government's policy in the 1930s of promoting the minority Tutsi as the ruling elite over the impoverished Hutu majority. A growing "Hutu Power" movement led to increasing tensions between the Hutu and Tutsi, with the minority Tutsi coming increasingly under attack by the Hutu. A series of conflicts drove many Tutsi out of Rwanda and into Uganda. In October 1990, the Tutsi-led RPF attempted to fight their way back into Rwanda. In 1993, the internationally negotiated Arusha Accords (so named because they were negotiated in Arusha, Tanzania) established a power-sharing agreement between the Hutu government and the RPF. Despite the leadership of President Juvénal Habyarimana, a moderate Hutu, the extremist drive to eliminate the Tutsi "cockroaches" grew. In opposition to the Arusha Accords, radical Hutus promoted a campaign that called for the extermination of the Tutsi.

On April 6, 1994, an airplane carrying the presidents of Rwanda and Burundi was shot down as it landed in Kigali, the capital of Rwanda. The assassinations were believed to be the work of Hutu extremists. This event reignited tensions and touched off an orchestrated genocidal campaign by Hutu Interahamwe ("those who fight together") that meant to murder all Tutsis and moderate Hutus. During a one-hundred-day period from April 7 to mid-July 1994, an estimated 1 million Rwandans were systematically slaughtered. Most victims were killed with machetes or farm tools in one of the most gruesome events of our time.

In the weeks and days leading up to the genocide, Lieutenant-General Roméo Dallaire, the Canadian officer in command of the United Nations Assistance Mission in Rwanda (UNAMIR), the peacekeeping force initially tasked with implementing the Arusha Accords, saw the signs of the impending attack. As the genocide started, Dallaire attempted to seize weapons landing in Kigali and pleaded for military support, but the United States and the United Nations refused. Dallaire's force heroically protected several groups of Tutsis and moderate Hutus from attack, but could not stop the wider killing. CIA intelligence briefing documents would later show that the US officials had known of the "final solution to eliminate all Tutsis" and did not act, largely out of fear of another engagement like Somalia. President Clinton would later reflect that if the United States had acted earlier, at least a third of those killed might have been saved.[1]

As the genocide escalated, the Tutsi-led RPF rapidly pushed into the country from neighboring Uganda. Many Rwandan Hutus, including the Hutu Interahamwe perpetrators, were displaced. Over 2.1 million Rwandans crossed into neighboring Tanzania, Burundi, and Zaire (now the Democratic Republic of the Congo), creating an unprecedented humanitarian crisis. UN agencies, including the UN High Commission for Refugees (UNHCR) and UNICEF, partnered with large NGOs like Médecins Sans Frontières, CARE, and Save the Children to establish an aid system for the massive camps. In May 1994, I arrived at the refugee camp in Ngara, Tanzania, just across the border from Rwanda, as more refugees were streaming in. Aid agencies were also arriving daily, and the UNHCR was struggling to coordinate all of the new actors. After meeting with representatives of the UN and a few NGOs that intended to set up relief operations, I walked around the camp and among the refugees, met with NGO field staff, and made my way to the bridge over Rusumo Falls, which separates Tanzania from Rwanda. As I stood on the bridge and looked down, I could see the bloated bodies that had been dumped into the river in Rwanda and floated downstream. It was a horrific sight. The bodies had gathered in the eddies by the falls, bleached and bloated from exposure to the hot sun. The image is seared into my memory even today.

I turned back to look at the vast camp. It was truly overwhelming: with nearly a half-million people here in Ngara and another million crossing into Goma, Zaire, the need was unimaginable. A haze from thousands of cooking fires hung over the camp, where countless refugees walked along the winding mud paths between tiny makeshift plastic and branch shelters that went on as far as I could see. We wanted to help, but the camps were chaotic, and there were dozens of organizations trying to work and more coming every day. We decided to leave and try to make our way into Rwanda itself, to rebuild medical care in the devastated country.

Meanwhile, the refugee camps in Tanzania and Zaire grew increasingly dangerous. In Goma, nearly 1 million Rwandan refugees settled on the volcanic savannah. There was no reasonable access to sanitation, and the soil could not drain the massive amount of human waste. NGOs and UN agencies struggled to provide basic necessities. The nearby lake, the main source of water for the camps, became polluted with fecal material. In July 1994, a cholera epidemic struck Goma. The mortality rates were staggering, with over 40,000 refugees dying in three weeks. The international aid community struggled to address the needs for cholera treatment, access to clean water, and disposal of thousands of the dead, but relief efforts proved insufficient for many reasons. The scale-up required to manage the epidemic was beyond any organization's capacity, a challenge compounded by the deteriorating security conditions in the massive camp. The encampment was a breeding ground for not only disease, but also violence. Thousands of Hutu extremists were organizing within the camp, re-arming and planning a counterattack into Rwanda. Security deteriorated, and many more Tutsis were murdered. Several NGOs, including Doctors Without Borders, left the camps because of dangerous conditions and lack of a political solution for creating a stable setting.

Shortly after, I went with Ken Isaacs and his team from Samaritan's Purse to Kigali, where very few aid agencies had arrived. The scene was apocalyptic. There were still remnents of bodies along the roads, ditches, and fields, with arms and legs strewn about like parts of mannequins. It was there that we met Lieutenant Colonel Rose Kabuye, a tall, thin Rwandan woman with a powerful presence who would later become the mayor of Kigali. She gave our team permission to work and to use a compound in Kigali as our home and headquarters, encouraging us to rebuild the Central Hospital of Kigali (CHK).

We set about the task of rebuilding CHK, a 400-bed referral hospital in the middle of the capital where hundreds had been murdered. The RPF had removed the dead and buried them in a mass grave on the hospital grounds, but it was common to find limbs and body parts that had not been buried or had been dug up by dogs. Every room was destroyed and looted, desks overturned and smashed, and paper medical records strewn across the empty corridors. One of the rooms was full of flies, and a black, gelatinized coating of blood covered the floor, while the walls were covered with a fine mist of blood. The grounds of the once-busy hospital were like a ghost town. There were no patients, and the few remaining staff who had returned had gone to the UN medical compound, away from the main facility. It was one of the darkest and most disturbing settings in which I've ever worked, and everywhere I turned was another grim reminder of the terrible events that had occurred just weeks before.

I worked with several colleagues to reestablish surgical services, the emergency department, in-patient medical beds, and a functional administration of the entire hospital. We formed a mirror administration that paired a Rwandan hospital leader with an expatriate counterpart, so the hospital director, nursing director, and administrative team all had an American counterpart to help them recreate a leadership and management system for the facility. The hospital compound was rebuilt, ward by ward. Before too long, CHK was once again the central referral center for Kigali.

One morning, while I worked in the emergency room, a young boy was brought in with a small laceration to his leg. He had cut it on a piece of wire while climbing a fence. The wound was minor and would only take a few stitches to close, but the boy was hysterical. He was screaming and thrashing and crying inconsolably, not letting any of us near him. Through our nurse interpreter, I asked his caregiver, his uncle, who had brought him from an orphanage, why he was so distraught. He told me that during the genocide a few months before, Hutu militia had combed through the boy's village and murdered his entire family with machetes. In the struggle the boy was struck on the head and left to die in a ditch, atop a pile of others from his village. He lay motionless on a bed of corpses all day, pretending to be dead, until the militia had finished with the village and left. He then snuck out and found his way to a refugee camp, alone. He had hardly spoken since.

I could hardly contemplate the tragedy he had experienced. I could only eventually sew his wound and send him back home with his uncle. His was only one of hundreds of thousands of horrific stories from the genocide, each equally tragic, each intensely personal. As a health worker, I had to focus on the concrete tasks of rebuilding the hospital and managing patients in the ER, and after a time, I really couldn't listen to any more stories. I knew that they would follow me home. I finally stopped wanting to know any more and stepped back to just do the work. My retreat to simply providing clinical care was my only means of self-preservation.

The horrors of the genocide affected everyone who worked in Rwanda and in the surrounding camps. The struggles of aid agencies in the aftermath of the genocide also upended the relief community permanently. In 1996, a pivotal report, the *Joint Evaluation of Emergency Assistance in Rwanda,* declared that lack of coordination and universal standards had contributed to the high mortality rates among Rwandan refugees.[2] The experiences of many relief agencies in Rwanda, and the findings of this report, created a groundswell of activism within the aid world. A solidarity of purpose emerged among aid agencies: to create new systems to better coordinate humanitarian aid, and to standardize and make accountable the delivery of emergency relief. One of the most important outcomes of this post-Rwanda reckoning was the Sphere Project.

Spearheaded by the International Federation of the Red Cross and Red Crescent (IFRC), the Sphere Project, a field guide on humanitarian standards, focused on two major principles. The first was the notion that refugees and threatened communities have rights, including the right to receive aid, and that aid organizations have a duty to provide that aid. The second principle was that aid must be standardized and provided in a consistent, responsible manner. Sphere promoted standards in the various sectors of humanitarian service, including food, water, sanitation, shelter, health, and security, and provided concrete guidance on what services were to be provided, to whom, and to what extent. Sphere was adopted by several hundred NGOs, and today, several updates later, it guides aid agencies in providing more appropriate, effective, and principled humanitarian relief. Both directly and symbolically, Sphere represented a dramatic change in the scope and responsibility of aid agencies. Aid was no longer just focused on moving around bags of rice and boxes of medicine; it had become a tool of diplomacy.

Sphere also ushered in a new era of professionalism. The field of emergency humanitarian aid was increasingly understood as unique and distinct from development work. Humanitarian relief was emerging as its own field, with unique environments, technical challenges, and required expertise. Individuals and organizations that performed well in these complex environments were not necessarily the same as those that undertook long-term relief efforts. The skills required to effectively manage workforce, supply chain, and long-term developmental efforts were very different from those required for the rapid deployment of aid efforts in insecure political settings. Humanitarian aid workers were trained in negotiating access, scaling up services rapidly, and working in the dynamic environments of war and disaster.

When I returned home from Rwanda to the emergency department in Chicago, the similarities of my two fields became even more evident. Just as the aid community was developing its skills, practices, and standards, emergency medicine was further developing as a field distinct from general medicine and other specialties, and establishing itself as a medical safety net for the community. Emergency humanitarian relief indeed seemed to be the "emergency medicine" of the larger global health field. As I stood with one foot in each world, I turned to the lessons learned from the growing field of emergency medicine to guide the development of the nascent field of humanitarian relief.

In the 1980s and 1990s, medical care in the United States began shifting toward a model of evidence-based care, a movement to translate clinical research into improved patient care. This had direct implications for the humanitarian aid field, in which rigorous research was lacking. If humanitarian assistance was to emerge as a respected profession, it needed a unique and discrete base of evidence to inform the work of aid providers. While the field had several excellent researchers, including senior epidemiologists Ron Waldman, Michael Toole, and Les Roberts, there were no dedicated centers for high-quality research of practical issues in humanitarian aid. Furthermore, the research that was being done was generally not used by aid agencies to change their practice. The aid world needed more and better research, and more and better ways to make these findings available to the agencies in the field.

The second gap that I saw was the lack of a professional pathway for aid providers. For humanitarian aid to become a specialized field with experts trained in aid provision, there had to be a clear career path. This needed to include, I believed, formal undergraduate and graduate studies in humanitarian response, and curricula in major universities that would advance the idea of humanitarian assistance as a science and profession, as well as provide nuanced training for existing humanitarian practitioners.

In order to push this agenda forward, I decided to combine my growing field experience with a better understanding of public health. I enrolled in a summer program at the Harvard School of Public Health and completed my Masters of Public Health degree at the University of Illinois, doing most of my coursework remotely from Rwanda. I also established the first international emergency medicine fellowship in 1996 as a way to help young physicians integrate global health and emergency medicine and build their ability to lead relief efforts. My first fellow, David Townes, would go on to work as a medical epidemiologist for the CDC and as a public health expert for the US Office of Foreign Disaster Assistance. There are now twenty-six international emergency medicine fellowships in the United States.

I also realized that I needed to be in a place with deep expertise in international public health. In 1997, I took a faculty position at Johns Hopkins University in Baltimore, where I would serve as an emergency physician at the Johns Hopkins Hospital and teach courses at the Johns Hopkins School of Public Health. Hopkins was a unique and powerful place, and one that would prove crucial in lighting the path before me. First, it was home to one of the earliest and most important emergency medicine programs in the United States. The chairman of that department, Gabe Kelen, had established a strong research program that was making research a credible and important part of the field of emergency medicine. Johns Hopkins Hospital was the best in the nation and set national and international standards in what academic emergency medicine should look like. Likewise, the Johns Hopkins School of Public Health was the largest and among the most important schools of its kind in the world. More ministers of health had trained at Hopkins than at any other school, and the name was well known throughout the global health world.

This position allowed me to be a part of the growing field of emergency medicine and to form my own ideas about humanitarian professionalism in a stimulating academic environment. I wanted to apply the lessons learned in building the new medical specialty of emergency medicine to the new, dynamic, and somewhat-unpredictable field of humanitarian aid. I hoped to work with some of the finest researchers in the field. A public health colleague, Gilbert Burnham, was already running excellent training programs for practitioners in humanitarian assistance, and together we began building a larger academic identity within the aid community. My colleagues at the Johns Hopkins School of Public Health were not only talented researchers, but they were also deeply experienced in the field. They demonstrated a principle that guides me to this day: to create a close link to aid agencies, academics must be deeply engaged in the field. In our collective work, I could see the model of academic partnerships with NGOs and the United Nations as a way to push the field forward in a smarter, more evidence-based way.

After arriving at Hopkins, I resumed the balancing act of going on overseas missions and returning to clinical work in the ER. Both were intense. The emergency department at Johns Hopkins cared for over 90,000 patients a year, most of them from the inner-city Baltimore "knife and gun club." The ER at Hopkins was busy, full of penetrating traumas, heroin addicts, and all manner of severe medical emergencies. The physicians, nurses, and staff consistently performed excellently, even under the crushing pace, and, as in the ERs I had encountered during my residency, we learned to depend on each other. Every emergency physician knows the feeling of being completely overwhelmed at 3:00 a.m. with yet another gunshot wound coming through the doors while the rest of the city sleeps. Nevertheless, Hopkins felt like the right place to be: always on duty, day or night.

My days in the ER were incredibly busy but also deeply fulfilling. Life at home became busier and more fulfilling as well. Julie and I had our first daughter, Alexandra, in 1996, followed by our son, Jackson, in 1998 and eventually our youngest, Isabella, in 2002. Julie completed her fellowship in urogynecology and pelvic surgery at Johns Hopkins and joined the faculty. This double-doctor family with three kids and a nanny spelled shorter deployments and a more stable lifestyle, but I still felt the pull of the field. My wonderful in-laws, Don and Kathy Arnold, never hesitated to load up their minivan and drive all the way from Champaign, Illinois, to Baltimore every time I had to travel abroad, often at very short notice. Julie remained a strong supporter and nurturing presence, and somehow I was able to maintain my dual career as an emergency physician and a humanitarian aid worker.

Teaching at the School of Public Health brought its own amazing rewards. I was surrounded by world-class faculty with deep field experience, and they were changing global public health. The Hopkins public health students were also a tremendous source of learning and growth.

Having an academic home base while working in the field provided some unique opportunities to involve my students in real-world events. One such opportunity centered on relief efforts mounted in response to the Kosovo War and the subsequent humanitarian crisis.

Kosovo was a province of Serbia that borders Albania to the West. Serbian political and social policies discriminating against the ethnic Albanians in Kosovo led to tensions before, during, and after the larger conflicts in the Balkans in the 1990s. In 1995, the Kosovo Liberation Army (KLA), composed largely of Albanian Kosovars, launched a series of military advances against the Serbian army with the aim of establishing Kosovo as an independent nation. The 1995 Dayton Agreement ended the Bosnian War, but the issue of Kosovo's bid for independence remained unresolved and drew little attention until the KLA attacked Serbian and Yugoslav security forces, leading to the first phase of the Kosovo War. Increasing violence led to NATO military intervention, including a bombing campaign intended to force Yugoslav troops to withdraw. Madeleine Albright, then the US Secretary of State, championed the NATO bombing in Kosovo, later noting that "what we did there was not legal, but it was right."[3] NATO's bombing campaign was one of the first times that a humanitarian and human rights goal—namely, the prevention of ethnic cleansing—drove military action. As the bombing increased, the Serbs stepped up their efforts to drive Kosovars out of Kosovo. During the conflict, over 11,000 died, and nearly a million ethnic Albanians fled Kosovo, traveling over the mountains into northern Albania. The UN High Commission for Refugees estimated that up to 25 percent of the entire population of Kosovo had fled. Refugees were crossing the mountainous border into Albania at the rate of 4,000 people per hour.

As the refugees started their migration, a number of large NGOs began to mobilize to build refugee camps in the small town of Hamallah. The Albanian authorities set aside large swaths of land for campsites. I once again received a call from colleagues from Samaritan's Purse, with whom I had worked in Somalia, Rwanda, and Bosnia. I was asked to fly to Tirana, Albania, and to make my way to Hamallah to design and build health services for a planned 30,000-refugee settlement. I agreed to deploy to Kosovo and made plans to leave within seventy-two hours. I would need a blueprint for comprehensive medical and public health services for refugees arriving within weeks.

At the time, I was teaching a class at Hopkins on humanitarian emergencies and public health crises. In our studies, we had been following the events of the Kosovo War and discussing its public health implications. After I received the call to deploy to the field, I made arrangements for another faculty member to cover my class for the next month and switched out of all of my emergency department shifts. Before I left, I met with all of my students and offered them a special assignment. Instead of writing a term paper, I asked them to design, in the following forty-eight hours, a comprehensive refugee health program specifically designed for the types of problems facing the Kosovar refugees crossing the border.

The entire class volunteered to help. I gave them a primer to aid them in modeling their proposed programs. They then divided up into small groups to develop plans for supply management, medical staffing, public health, sanitation, pharmaceuticals, minor and major surgical capacity, inpatient and outpatient medical, reproductive health, and a host of other issues. They did extensive background research and met on their own, staying up late into the night. By the time I left, my students had drafted a comprehensive plan for integrated medical services for three refugee camps with an expected population of 30,000. This was exactly the blueprint I needed.

I arrived, secured my Albanian medical license, and began work with the authorities to confirm and fund the plan. I felt like a kid who had come to a test with all of the answers. The plan my students had created highlighted some unique features of the situation. Many of the NGOs providing health services in the Kosovo crisis were basing their choice of medications and supplies on their experience in African refugee camps, which typically have high rates of malnutrition and communicable diseases like malaria, measles, and diarrheal illnesses like cholera. My students took the time to research the baseline health problems of the migrating Kosovars, including higher risks of hypertension, heart disease, and noncommunicable illnesses and low or nonexistent rates of chronic malnutrition, measles, or malaria. The types of providers, treatments, equipment, and pharmaceuticals needed would be entirely different because of the very different nature of the expected illnesses.

As the healthcare program in Albania developed and went into action, the full value of my students' plan became obvious. They had predicted it perfectly: the Kosovo refugees suffered from many illnesses and injuries, but those maladies were entirely different than those seen in Africa or Asia. Instead of malaria, we saw uncontrolled blood pressure. Instead of infant mortality, we saw ill elderly people. Instead of chronic malnutrition, we saw overwhelming fatigue. Through this exercise, we saved the organization from wasting resources, saved our refugee patients by having the right supplies at the right moment, and saved my students a term paper. This moment taught me the importance and power of evidence. The differences between the Kosovar and Sudanese refugees were obvious, but aid planning did not always have a way to account for such variance. The best evidence and the best predictors of population needs were often not readily available. These factors may seem simple, but for a massively complex undertaking like humanitarian aid, sometimes the big picture is the last thing to come into focus. This exercise with my students taught me the critical importance of using evidence to plan humanitarian intervention, and to measure what we do. It also taught me the power of inspiration. These students were not working all night to avoid a term paper; they were inspired by a real-world problem, and they worked together to solve it. There was no publication, no individual distinction, just the desire to contribute to something real. This was a lesson that I would carry with me for the next decades of my career.

5

IN THE FIELD

THE SOUND OF MASSIVE ANTONOV ENGINES ROARED in the sky above South Sudan. Staff, patients, and families scrambled for small bunkers, seeking shelter from the third air raid in two weeks. Stragglers scattered through the bush, running away from the raid's target, Lui Hospital—the latest of several civilian structures targeted by government forces in the North in their battle against the Sudanese People's Liberation Army (SPLA) in the South.

I had been outside, meeting with our medical assistants for a training session. We had gathered under a large mango tree to escape the sun. As we heard the Antonov, a Russian-made cargo plane, approaching, we gathered up several of the medical and nursing staff and ran toward the red-earth bunkers, simple trenches dug in the ground to shield us from shrapnel. Some hospital staff grabbed patients and huddled behind the cinderblock walls of the hospital, hoping there would not be a direct hit.

I crouched with five or six men and women, including a young child, all of us soaked with sweat, silently looking up at the sky. It was hot and claustrophobic, and everyone remained quiet, straining to hear if the sound was growing louder. Often the Antonovs would simply fly overhead without dropping any bombs, just to instill fear. That day, only one bomb was dropped. It exploded outside the village with a deep, percussive blast. A few minutes later, the hum of the engines grew faint, and we emerged from the bunkers to resume our day. The bomb had exploded in a field, injuring no one. Nevertheless, for the government forces, it was a successful mission. Their campaign of intimidation and fear reminded the villages of the South that they were always under threat and could never rest.

South Sudan is one of the poorest regions in the world, with a long history of conflict, economic vulnerability, and food insecurity. From the 1990s until today, Sudan has increasingly become dependent on food aid.[1] South Sudan also lacks adequate medical services. During my time in the country, the only reliable medical care in the region was provided by international NGOs. Starting in the late 1990s, several organizations set up operations in South Sudan, including Médecins Sans Frontières, the International Medical Corps, and Samaritan's Purse. Humanitarians managed various forms of medical and surgical care and formed the backbone of health programming in Sudan.

In 1997, an MSF facility near Lui closed down. To fill the gap, Samaritan's Purse set out to rebuild Lui Hospital. The hospital was built by Scottish missionary surgeon Kenneth Fraser, who had arrived in the 1920s in the isolated region of Eastern Equatoria in South Sudan, a regional slave-trading center in the 1800s. Lui Hospital had once served the entire region but was destroyed during the First Sudanese Civil War

(1955–1972). During the Second Sudanese Civil War (1983–2005), the hospital grounds were destroyed. The ruins became overgrown with brush. Paths nearby were marked with red skull-and-crossbones signs to keep people away from the buildings. The corrugated tin roofs had long since been stolen for scrap, and only cinderblock walls remained from the old hospital. Those walls were covered with charcoal drawings made by both North and South Sudanese soldiers as the hospital traded hands during the long second civil war. The sketches depicted tanks and other weapons, turning the old hospital into a strange chronicle of the conflict. Hiding beneath the scrub grass and overgrown weeds on the hospital grounds were another legacy of the war: scores of landmines.

The mines under the old hospital were below-the-ground anti-personnel blast mines. Known locally as "black widows," these small, simple devices were designed to maim. When triggered, the mine would explode and shred the foot and lower leg of the victim, often leading to his or her death and a halt to the military advance. Mines created a long-lived legacy of the conflict, outlasting the people who placed them. They remained buried and silent, and prevented any use of the land for farming, grazing, or building. Yellow caution tape and signs warned villagers to keep clear of the old hospital grounds. There were a few paths that had been de-mined, and if we took care to stay within their narrow limits, we could safely walk to the abandoned building.

To start the process of rebuilding the hospital, we hired a local mine removal expert named Morrison who had been trained by UNMAS, the United Nations Mine Action Service. A gregarious Sudanese man who had worked abroad for several years and had returned home to Lui to clear the hospital, he was in his early thirties, experienced and confident, and greeted me with a wide smile and a strong handshake. One morning, as he was showing me his plan for removing the mines around the hospital, he absentmindedly grabbed my hand and held it casually as we walked. Holding hands with a male friend while walking was a custom in Sudan, and though it seems strange to Westerners, it's a common gesture of friendly affection. He led me along, chattering about the area to be cleared, his hopes for the new hospital and what it would mean for his people, and his hope that one day South Sudan would be peaceful.

The work of de-mining was intense, slow, and extremely dangerous. Morrison and a crew of helpers carefully laid a grid across an area of the hospital property using stakes and red-and-white striped tape. Dressed in light-blue UN mine protection gear, they cleared small garden-sized plots by sweeping them with a metal detector and then painstakingly and delicately prodding the ground by poking a thin metal stick into the soil at a forty-five-degree angle. The light touch of the stick would reveal the presence of a mine without triggering the explosive device. Upon finding a mine, Morrison would expose and carefully remove it, take it to a pit in a field outside of the village, and detonate it. From time to time, we would hear the deep "thud" of exploding ordnance as Morrison disposed of another mine. Over the course of weeks, the hospital grounds started to become more habitable.

We set up a temporary medical clinic and operating room in a school across the dirt road from the hospital and met with the village elders to work out a partnership for redeveloping the property. Someone brought out a heavy old manual typewriter owned by the local pastor, and we typed up a contract between the NGO and the Diocese of Lui, the Episcopal church that owned the property. We celebrated the partnership with goat stew and fufu, a dough-like cassava paste ubiquitous in Sudanese cuisine. Over the next few months, the materials needed to de-mine, rebuild, and re-equip the hospital came in by plane and truck. The first surgeries were done by flashlight, and the first "ambulances" were Honda all-terrain vehicles that could travel over the rough land.

As the property was de-mined, we made plans to move our facility from the school to the hospital, which would still need a roof and windows. One day, while working in the operating room, I heard the boom of a detonated mine. It had become a familiar sound, and I didn't think anything of it. But a few minutes later, I heard screams and calls for help. On a walkthrough of the grounds, Morrison had triggered a mine that his sweep had missed. The explosion blew off one of his feet. He was rushed to the operating theater, where surgeon Bill Greiser and I looked at his wound. The foot was gone, and the lower leg around the ankle was shredded. Morrison gritted his teeth, delirious with pain.

We took him immediately into surgery, where he was given ketamine anesthesia. The destroyed bone, muscle, and tissue were cut back, creating a below-the-knee amputation. It was difficult to tell how much the blast injury had affected the leg, and we closely watched his condition. Later that night, Morrison developed shaking chills and worsening pain. He was taken back to the operating room, and the leg was amputated above the knee. Even with the second amputation, he steadily worsened, becoming delirious and combative. He died on the operating table the next day, felled by shock and overwhelming infection. The medical staff sat quietly on the rough benches outside of the operating room, exhausted and demoralized. I knew the people of Lui had heard about his death when I heard cries of mourning coming from all over the village. Morrison's family and the rest of the village came quietly to the hospital. They walked right by us, came to his bedside, and wept. They washed his body, then wrapped him in white muslin and carried him away, out of the hospital and into the bush. Although we felt that we had become a close part of the community, we were not invited to Morrison's burial. We were visitors, and this was their grief.

Some time later, I walked through the quiet future hospital, looking at where we would place the wards, operating rooms, and other departments. On one of the walls was written: "Morrison was here. He made this hospital safe for Lui."

The hospital grew quickly. As the only formal medical facility for a population of over 300,000 within a 160-kilometer radius, people would sometimes walk for two weeks to receive care from the international and local medical staff at Lui. This medical care was basic, even austere by Western standards, but it was the best in the region. Staffed by veteran surgeons like Warren Cooper, a physician I had trained with in Chicago, the hospital became a magnet for those fleeing the North–South conflict raging less than seventy kilometers away. In a short time, the tiny village of Lui swelled to an impromptu town of nearly 9,000.

The hospital was also a magnet for soldiers moving between the lines of battle. Although the facility was generally off-limits to soldiers (and, more importantly, to weapons), many times men returning from the front line, drunk on banana beer, would push their way into the compound. These fighters, who were SPLA soldiers from the region, brandished AK-47s and demanded food, medical supplies, or care for one of their injured comrades. While this was often an inconvenience, our ability to work safely in the area depended on our relationship with these armed groups, and we generally had a cooperative rapport with the militias.

Indeed, in much of my work in the field, gaining access to refugees and war-affected communities was less of a theoretical construct and more of a local, practical task. Gaining access was best accomplished by gaining trust, and much of gaining trust was developing a personal rapport with those in the communities where we worked. In South Sudan, many of these initial relationships were with the local militia, including the SPLA soldiers who occupied the area, and they proved to be crucial connections.

Even before we rebuilt the hospital in Lui, we had traveled to that region to scout out a suitable area to work. After our small plane, a Cessna Caravan, landed on a short dirt airstrip near the village of Maridi in Western Equatoria, we hired a truck and headed out to scope out the access points for the future hospital in Lui, farther north. As we drove northward, we encountered a group of SPLA soldiers who were manning a post along the (only) dirt road, close to the front line of the conflict with the North. The soldiers stopped the truck and made us get out. They surrounded us and began asking questions about why we were there. We explained that we were from a medical NGO hoping to rebuild a hospital farther north.

"Are you a doctor?" one of the soldiers asked.

I nodded yes.

"Come with me," he said and motioned for me to follow.

The group led me to a small, dark hut to see one of their fellow soldiers who had been shot in the wrist several weeks before. The wounded soldier's right wrist and hand were swollen to twice their normal size. I examined the wrist, which was obviously fractured and infected, and pus oozed from the site of the wound. The soldier was stoic but in obvious pain. I told them that I would do what I could to help. With the other soldiers gathered around, I pulled out a small surgical kit that I carried with me in the field, with a few instruments and some dressing material. After injecting the wound with lidocaine, a local anesthetic, I began to cut out the infected tissue with a scalpel. Beads of sweat were pouring from the soldier's forehead, but he stayed completely still. I drained nearly a cup of pus from the wound and extracted the bullet, which was of great interest to the twenty or so bystanders. I washed the wound out with water from my water bottle as best I could, placed a wick for drainage in it, and then splinted the fractured wrist. I handed him a bottle of antibiotic pills from the kit and gave him instructions through a translator to keep it clean and splinted.

Several months later, we came back to build the hospital and were again stopped at an SPLA checkpoint by soldiers who asked several questions about what we were carrying and where we were going. Again, they asked us to get out of the Land Cruiser and to stand by the roadside and wait. I wondered if this would be a recurrent problem for our future work. One of the men told me to stay where I was and called out to another. A group of heavily armed soldiers strode up and surrounded me.

"You're the doctor who came here before," one of them said through an interpreter.

I nodded. "Yes, I was here a few months ago."

He turned to his comrade, who held out his hand. He showed me his wrist, and I finally recognized him as the soldier I had treated months before. He broke into a broad grin. To my great relief, the wrist had healed beautifully, and he could move it around freely. He grabbed my hand and introduced me to the group of soldiers as his *"beny wal"*—wise—doctor. After several minutes of handshakes and greetings, most of which were unintelligible to me, he thanked me and motioned for us to go on through. We never had difficulty with a checkpoint again.

As the rebuilt hospital in Lui expanded, it also became a target for aerial attacks from the Northern government forces. The primary mode of attack was indiscriminant bombing by the Antonov, a lumbering plane that flies far too high to allow for accurate bombing. The crude, cheaply made barrel bombs used by the government forces were filled with scrap metal, sharp objects, and explosives. The crew would simply push the bombs out of the plane's back cargo bay mid-flight. Their targets were civilian communities. On impact, the barrel bombs propelled a hail of deadly shrapnel in all directions. The government bombing raids had no military targets; their goal was to instill fear and panic in the villages below. At Lui, when the roar of Antonovs rose in the distance, all work ceased. People scrambled for the roughly dug bomb shelters as the planes soared overhead. Even without dropping bombs, their looming presence forced the hospital staff and patients to evacuate and run for shelter, disrupting all medical and surgical care.

My colleagues and I had flown over the green savannah of Lui many times in the past. We realized that the hospital's silver corrugated tin roof made it a perfect target, especially with the red cross emblazoned on it. I felt that something less obvious might be safer for our patients and staff, so I hired several Sudanese workers to paint the roof green. When the shipment of paint arrived, the workers came to the hospital in the early morning to start the job. They began brushing the forest-green oil paint on the tin roof, but by mid-morning, they came down. I asked when they would resume their work.

"It's too hot, brother," they called back from the shade of a mango tree.

"It's not too hot to get bombed," I replied. "C'mon, we need to finish this."

They smiled and shrugged their shoulders. "Maybe a little more tomorrow."

I was impatient. I would only be in Lui for a couple more weeks and wanted to see the painting done. Sure that a green roof would hide us from further attack, I decided to do it myself, and a friend and I climbed up. It was blazing hot, and we were aware that we were roasting up on the shiny metal roof. But after several hours in the hot equatorial sun, we had painted all of the tin green. I proudly came down, only to be greeted by pointing and laughter. I was lobster-red, already blistering from the worst sunburn of my life. My red skin became quite the curiosity around the village, and several of the young Sudanese boys would follow me to point and laugh. The young boys had a habit of taking handfuls of motor oil and rubbing it on their skin till it glistened pitch black in the sun. They suggested that next time I try the same method to prevent sunburn. That evening found me shaking from a fever in my bed, too sore to move and too embarrassed to complain.

I was wrong about the effectiveness of the green paint. Despite the roof camouflage, the terror of the bombers continued. In 1999, North Sudan expanded its aerial campaign against the South, dropping over 400 bombs in more than sixty attacks. NGOs and UN agencies continued to protest these attacks as clear breaches of international humanitarian law and the Geneva Conventions. On March 6, 2000, President Clinton's special envoy to Sudan, Harry Johnston, visited Khartoum, the capital of the North, for the first time. During that visit, the bombings in the South escalated. Several bombs hit Lui Hospital, killing nine people, injuring dozens, and badly damaging the hospital itself.

Sudan was just one casualty in a growing phenomenon: attacks on hospitals, medical staff, and the civilians they serve. Aid agencies and humanitarian medical staff worked in increasingly dangerous "asymmetrical" war zones. The concept of asymmetrical conflict grew out of the Afghan resistance to Soviet invasion in the 1980s. Such conflicts were fought between groups with uneven capabilities, such as terrorist groups fighting to overthrow government forces. Weaker parties in an asymmetric conflict use strategies such as embedding themselves within civilian communities. They use terror tactics to control populations, gain public support, and challenge larger, more powerful armies. The resistance posed by the Afghan mujahedeen, aided by US support as a form of proxy war, frustrated the Red Army and eventually led to the defeat of the Soviets. The success of the Afghan resistance contributed in part to the eventual collapse of the USSR.

As the Cold War ended, the number of interstate wars declined. Such traditional wars—one national government versus another—were replaced by a growing number of extremely violent intrastate conflicts that were, by definition, asymmetrical. The Sri Lankan civil war, which finally ended in 2009 after sixteen years of conflict, pitted the government of Sri Lanka against the Tigers of Tamil Eelam. The Tamil Tigers used guerilla warfare, suicide bombings, kamikaze-type attacks, and widespread terrorist tactics on civilian targets to disrupt every aspect of life under the Sri Lankan government. The most persistent asymmetrical conflict has been the long-term struggle between Israel and Palestinian armed groups such as Hamas. In this conflict, the highly trained, highly organized Israeli army mounts large military operations, using armored vehicles and air support, while the smaller, more poorly equipped Hamas and Palestinian Islamic Jihad forces use tactics such as cross-border shootings, checkpoint attacks, suicide bombings, and embedding themselves into the civilian population.

This last tactic makes asymmetrical conflict a major challenge for aid providers and humanitarians. All wars generate refugees and create health risks. But the use of civilian populations as a shield by combatants blurs these distinctions and brings innocent, unprotected groups into the line of fire. Aid agencies operating in asymmetrical conflicts find themselves working alongside the very militias that perpetuate these conflicts. Humanitarians are unarmed and form bonds with the communities they serve, largely depending on the goodwill and protection of local partners for their safety. In settings such as Sudan, this connection between locals and aid providers can give the appearance of complicity with rebel activities.

In such situations, hospitals and medical staff may no longer be seen as neutral, but may come to be viewed as participants in the conflict and supporters of the rebel movement. This loss of (perceived) neutrality can equate to a loss of safety. As asymmetrical conflicts have increased, attacks on medical aid workers have risen at an alarming rate. In the past twenty-five years, more than 1,000 aid workers have been killed in humanitarian settings. Many of these were health workers from organizations like the ICRC and MSF. Most of these attacks were deliberate assaults on aid workers with the goal of intimidation, disruption of services, or revenge.

South Sudan was one such place where militias blended into the civilian community. In fact, it was nearly impossible to separate the two groups. This blurring of military and civilian worlds would test my own sense of practical medical ethics.

One afternoon, while working in Lui Hospital, a short-wave radio message came in from Tindalo, a small village just northwest of Juba, on the front line of the conflict. The radio reported that several civilians had been injured in a battle near Tindalo, and that there was no way to evacuate the wounded. We loaded the Toyota Land Cruiser with medical supplies and headed to the front. The seventy-kilometer trip took three hours. Even in a rugged SUV, we had difficulty picking our way through the mud and brush on the two-track road. The red mud was as slippery as ice in some areas, and we spent much of the three hours outside of the truck, packing rocks under the tires for traction and pushing the vehicle out of ruts and gullies. By the time Ken Isaacs and I arrived at the site of the recent fighting, the sun was setting and we were covered in mud. We were greeted by the SPLA commander, who sat in a worn folding chair in the middle of a clearing, holding a radio and a small baton. Soldiers moved around the clearing, gathering up supplies.

"Where are the wounded?" I asked the commander. "Where are all the people from the village?"

"They are gone," he said.

He told me they had been carried off into the bush and pointed in a general direction where there was no road, only a few footpaths. The area had previously been mined, and I was advised by the soldiers not to try the paths, especially not in the waning light of the day. We had driven several hours to reach the wounded villagers, but now there were no civilians to evacuate. The commander lifted his baton toward his men.

"There are your wounded," he said.

I looked over the soldiers strewn across the clearing. They wore only parts of uniforms: a torn green shirt, a green bandana, ripped green shorts. Some wore flip-flop sandals instead of boots. All were dirty, sweaty, and gaunt. Kalashnikovs and RPGs lay against logs and trees, and a fire smoked nearby. Several of the soldiers were Dinkas, one of the largest ethnic groups in Sudan. The faces of the Dinka soldiers bore decorative scars, three cuts in the shape of a "V" along the forehead, ritually cut by the village elders with a thorn or a small knife once the boys reached adolescence. The markings gave them a striking, somewhat intimidating appearance.

I realized I could not reach the civilian casualties. I also realized that, as a physician, I could not just leave these injured soldiers behind. I discussed the issue with Ken and together we decided to treat the wounded fighters on site and evacuate those who needed immediate surgery. It was nearly dark when I spread a large blue plastic tarp on the ground and opened up a trunk of medical supplies. I had only basic equipment, not enough for any complicated procedures. I found a man who could translate and set out to find out what needed to be done. Over the next two hours, I treated injured soldiers in the clearing under the light of a flashlight.

The first man had a gunshot wound to the hip. He was in severe pain, but remained incredibly stoic. As I pulled his pants down, he looked straight ahead without saying a word, sweat pouring from his forehead. A few of his friends laughed as I pulled his clothes away to look at the wound, but they knew their comrade was seriously injured. A bullet had struck near the hip joint, but the resulting wound didn't appear to involve the pelvis, abdomen, or any of the leg's large blood vessels. I cleaned the wound with a mixture of water and betadine, packed it with gauze, and dressed it. Through the translator, I explained that we would take the soldier to the hospital that evening, as his wound would require proper debridement and possibly an operation. Next came a young solider with a penetrating abdominal wound. He was in early shock and required IV fluids and immediate transport back to the hospital for surgery. The young man was scared and shaking, and his comrades did not joke with him; they all thought he might die from his injury. I simply dressed his wound, gave him a dose of morphine, and carried him to the back of the Toyota.

There were a few others with minor injuries. One was a young man with a bullet wound to the arm. The bullet didn't seem to have penetrated the bone or any major vessels, and he also appeared stable. He could wait to be treated at the hospital later. I instructed one of his fellow soldiers to flush the wound with water using a syringe and then to bandage it. I fashioned a splint and sling and told the soldier to get to the hospital in the next few days.

Before leaving, I again asked the commander how I might find any injured civilians caught in the crossfire of the recent battle. He shrugged and said they were gone. We packed up our gear and the injured soldiers and began the journey back. The return trip was even worse than our earlier drive, with the glaze of red mud nearly impossible to drive through, even in a four-wheel-drive Land Cruiser. We got stuck repeatedly, sliding off the road and getting buried in mud ruts. It took almost four excruciating hours to get the injured men to the Lui Hospital compound, but we did finally arrive, and both soldiers not only survived to make it to the operating room, but eventually recovered.

The work in Sudan was intense and very different from work at home. There was no electricity and only the bare minimum of medical supplies. When not on duty, there was nothing to do after sunset except walk around the small village or read under the glow of a lantern. Nevertheless, I enjoyed my time there, and my colleagues, immensely. While on mission in Lui, I was joined by Tim Erickson, a longtime friend and fellow ER physician who had come to Sudan as part of a training program to transition SPLA soldiers to civilian medical assistants. During the training, we conducted a series of lectures, class discussions, and skill stations under a large mango tree. We used freshly killed goats to practice setting bones, suturing, and other procedures. Following the day of training, we skinned the well-sutured goat and had a barbecue for the evening dinner, a rare break from the normal beans and rice.

One evening, as we chatted in the waning light of dusk, the weather seemed to change dramatically. Instead of the usual warm, dry evening air, heavy thunderclouds moved in. The air became heavy and humid, as if it were about to pour. Walking along the path between the latrine and my *tukel* (the mud hut with a thatched roof where I slept), I noticed that the ground seemed to be crawling. When I shined my flashlight off the path onto the sparse scrub grass, I saw scorpions and tarantulas crawling everywhere. They were coming out of the ground in anticipation of the storm, and there were hundreds of them.

Tim and I immediately reverted to being teenagers. We ran around with coffee cans, collecting scorpions and spiders and comparing what we found. I grabbed a tarantula and tossed it at Tim, who caught it and threw it back like a hot potato. Tim was also a medical toxicologist with expertise on spider and snake poisonings, so he knew which creatures we could safely pick up. We collected dozens of tarantulas, snakes, and scorpions, pouring them onto the dinner table to inspect. After chasing the staff around with creatures, we finally released our temporary pets into the brush (far away from the hospital) and retreated to bed. I carefully tucked my gear into a duffel bag to discourage any unwanted guests. As I lay on my cot under the mosquito netting, I wondered what creatures might be in my hut. I shone my flashlight above me. Several tarantulas were perched on the net just above my head, having dropped from the thatched ceiling above. I was too exhausted to get out of bed and decided that I would simply ignore them, although I did tuck in the mosquito netting a bit more thoroughly than usual. I slept surprisingly well that night.

Coming home from a mission like Sudan was sometimes difficult. The world at home had moved forward without me, and there was no way to gently ease myself back into it. The emergency department pulled at me, always with a backlog of ER shifts and other responsibilities. My young kids were understandably eager to spend time with Dad, and my wife, weary from weeks of solo parenting, needed me. Even as I dove headfirst into normal life at home, I felt guilty about leaving my friends, colleagues, and patients in the field while I returned to the comforts of home. I wondered whether I should have or could have stayed longer, done more. But there was no time to brood on the decision, no time for reflection or soul searching. Eventually, I understood that these rapid transitions helped me readjust back to normal life. Dwelling too much on what I had just seen and done required time I did not have. Gradually, the issues that had been so critically important in Sudan grew further away and were replaced with the priorities of home and work, although I often would still feel dissatisfied that I had not done more.

After the first years of work abroad, I rarely spoke about my experiences in the field with friends or family. I would tell stories (like the night of the tarantulas) but would never really open up about the medical work, or the human suffering, or the frustrations. The context was so foreign to most people, and the emotions of being there were difficult to describe. I developed a habit of speaking very briefly about what I had been doing and not truly sharing the strange, gratifying, heartbreaking nature of practicing medicine in a distant war zone. The empathy I felt for my patients and my team in the field left me with a feeling of guilt as I returned to the stability of home. I found it difficult to reconcile the extreme poverty and vulnerability I witnessed abroad with the excesses of life in the United States.

Yet it was that sense of empathy that first drove me to become a doctor and humanitarian. The importance of understanding how other people feel was a strong part of my early religious upbringing and a theme that resonated through my childhood experiences. My father's stories of his confinement at Bergen-Belsen, the early death of my mother, and my medical training in inner-city Detroit all stimulated a deep sense of responsibility for those who suffer. I wanted to place myself in patients' shoes, to feel their needs and struggle with their problems. Empathy also powered the transformative moment when I witnessed the rescue of the young man trapped under a tractor. The injured boy was my age, and I felt his fear and vulnerability. Sharing in his helplessness, I resolved to be the one to help. Empathy remained a driving force in my subsequent education and residency. As I entered the aid world, it likewise compelled me to understand the terrible plight of the Somali woman in the refugee camp, and to realize my own limitations.

But empathy is not without peril. In emergency medicine, empathy can create anxiety for physicians. Caregivers can lose their bearings if they are completely inside the urgency of a crashing patient, the expressions of pain and fear. In the humanitarian field, that anxiety can be compounded by personal danger and the crushing needs of thousands of refugees. Empathy, I came to believe, was driving our compassion as aid workers. But it was also preventing humanitarians—including me—from stepping out of the immediacy of need to grasp the bigger picture. To be the one who helps on the scale of a humanitarian crisis, I needed a more objective, scientific view. I began to better understand this struggle early in my time at Johns Hopkins.

Sir William Osler, the founder of modern medicine, figures prominently in the medical culture of Johns Hopkins. Osler, a Canadian, began his career at Montreal's McGill University and eventually moved to the University of Pennsylvania in 1885. Four years later, he left Penn to become the first physician-in-chief of the new Johns Hopkins Hospital in Baltimore. But Osler did not merely practice medicine at Hopkins; he was also instrumental in the creation of the Johns Hopkins School of Medicine and became one of its first professors. He created the modern concept of residency training, which brought medical students out of the classroom and to the bedside for clinical education. The term "rounds" refers to the path Osler and his students took through the circular hallway under the dome of the original hospital at Hopkins as they saw patients and reviewed their care.

Before Osler left the University of Pennsylvania, he delivered a valedictory address that became the basis of his most famous essay, entitled "Aequanimitas." In a paper that has become a key document in the history of medicine, Osler urged the new generation of physicians to develop the virtue of equanimity: a sense of imperturbability and "a judicious measure of obtuseness." To Osler, calmness and coolness were essential qualities for a physician, even and especially under the most difficult circumstances. He suggested that physicians cultivate a degree of detachment, as some degree of distance was necessary for a physician to be effective. Dispassionate, rational decision-making could even instill confidence in a frightened patient.

While this notion of equanimity can conflict with the sense of empathy that drives many, including me, into medicine in the first place, equanimity has powerful applications in the humanitarian field. Creating more measurable, balanced, and evidence-driven humanitarian aid requires a significant measure of objectivity and even a sense of distance. To me, equanimity meant applying a more analytic perspective to the humanitarian aid world. This outlook led me to envision some of the fundamental changes necessary to transform aid into a profession.

I found that the best approach to thinking through my experiences providing aid in Sudan and elsewhere was to weave them into the courses I taught at Johns Hopkins. Preparing for and teaching class became my way of processing my experiences, explaining my frustrations, and sharing my satisfactions. The classroom became a place to reflect on the groundwork that we had laid in a larger context, and to be self-critical in a constructive way. With my students as collaborators, I could explore what I felt humanitarians were doing right, what we were doing wrong, and how we could better prepare to work in these new and dangerous environments. Teaching became a form of therapy for me.

Teaching also served as a way to step back and examine the larger issues affecting the aid community. I was experiencing in the field a small sample of the humanitarian world. I could see that the demands on aid providers were growing, and that the need for professionalism and leadership in this emerging field was growing as well. I had come to Johns

Hopkins because I saw that humanitarian aid was indeed its own unique discipline, very different from long-term development work in stable political settings. The number of aid agencies was growing, but there was no professional pathway for these new humanitarians. It was also clear to me that the world did not need more NGOs or UN agencies, but organizations to teach and professionalize aid workers. We needed a home for research, training, and innovation in humanitarian aid.

As I continued my work at Johns Hopkins, splitting my time between the ER and the disaster center at the School of Public Health, traveling abroad nearly every month became increasingly untenable. I very much needed to remain in both worlds—academic medicine and humanitarian assistance—but I also needed to be in the same place for more than a few months at a time. My solution to this problem was to create an academic program at Hopkins that could explore the changing landscape of aid and create new ways to engage with NGOs and the United Nations.

For help with such a large undertaking, I turned to Skip Burkle. A retired Navy captain, veteran military humanitarian, and one of the leading scholars on civil–military humanitarian affairs, Skip had led missions around the world. His résumé spanned 1975's Operation Baby Lift in Saigon to the 1991 Persian Gulf War, where he was the senior medical officer for the Al Khanjar Navy-Marine Trauma Center, the largest-ever Marine Corps field hospital built to serve forward troops in Operation Desert Storm. Skip was a great friend and mentor, and he would serve as one of my key academic collaborators for many years. He clearly saw the need to professionalize the next generation of humanitarian aid workers. To that end, he helped create a foundation for advancing aid through academics. The goal of the foundation was to apply science to the world of humanitarianism through new courses, new research, and new ways of collaborating across agencies.

My work in emergency medicine provided me with a unique perspective on how medicine and public health could inform humanitarian aid. I worked closely with Skip and public health experts like Gilbert Burnham, Ron Waldman, and Les Roberts, all leaders in applying rigorous research methods to the complex terrain of emergencies. The goals of their research were no longer theoretical, but aimed to transform the work of UN agencies and NGOs. This work advanced new ideas and new methods for improving relief. The next generation of aid leaders in the field would need to use research to understand the political, social, and legal dimensions of humanitarian assistance in order to take relief efforts to more dangerous, less secure settings.

Just as the humanitarian aid community seemed to have caught up to the challenges of the 1990s, the world changed. The attacks of September 11, 2001, created a new world order and brought a new set of challenges for international diplomacy, military intervention, and humanitarian response. The growing threat of Islamic extremism and the further erosion of humanitarian neutrality permanently altered the landscape for delivering assistance in many regions of the world. An ever-increasing number of crises were dominating the political landscape, and many countries were no longer safe for aid workers.

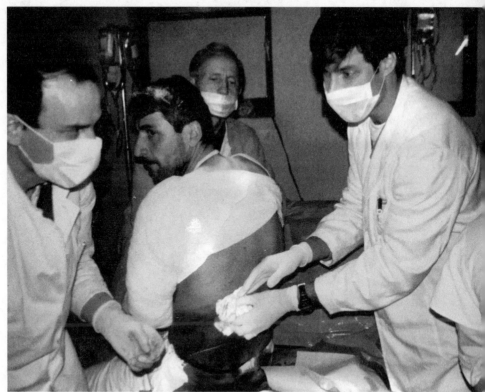

Placing a chest tube in a gun-shot wound patient, Bosnia, 1993. (Photograph by Michael VanRooyen)

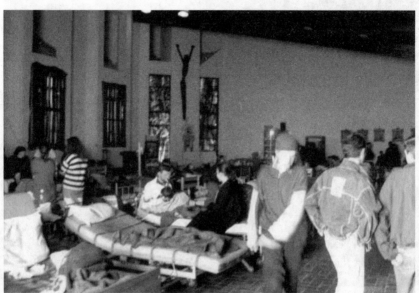

Nova Bila Hospital for the War Wounded (Fra. Mato Nikolić Hospital), 1993. (Photograph by Michael VanRooyen)

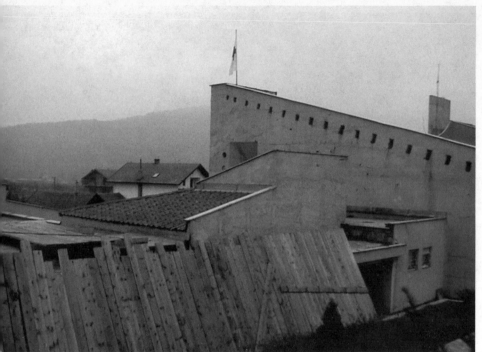

Exterior, Nova Bila Hospital for the War Wounded (Fra. Mato Nikolić Hospital), 1993. (Photograph by Michael VanRooyen)

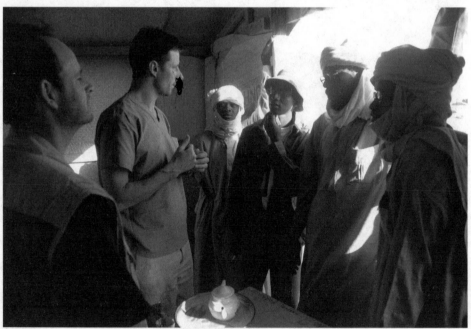

Talking with leaders in Kashuni Camp, Chad, 2005. (Photograph courtesy of Michael Wadleigh/ Gritty.org)

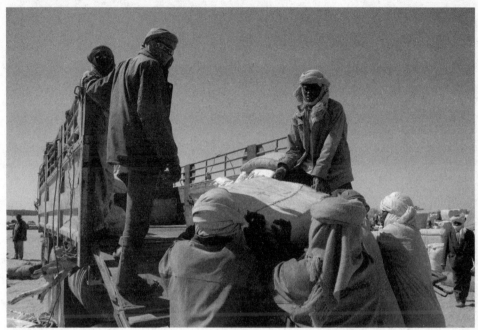

Food relief in Kashuni Camp, Chad, 2005. (Photograph courtesy of Michael Wadleigh/Gritty.org)

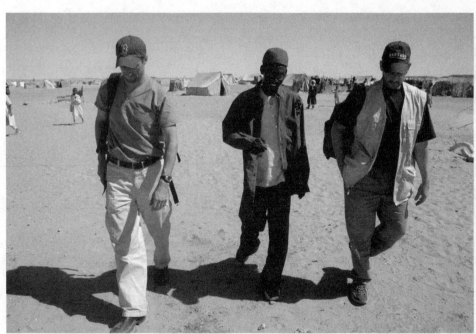

Team walking in Kashuni Camp, Chad, 2005. (Photograph courtesy of Michael Wadleigh/Gritty.org)

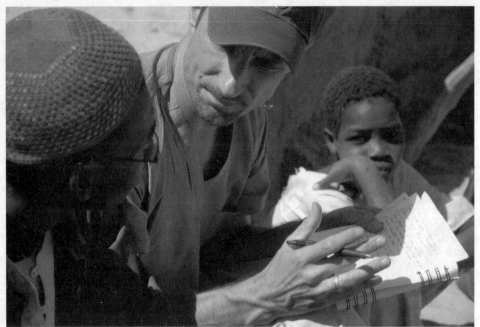

*Interviewing Darfuri refugees at Kashuni Camp, Chad, 2005. (Photograph courtesy of Michael Wadleigh/
Gritty.org)*

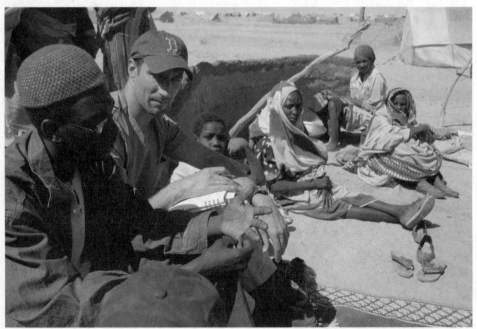

*Interviewing Darfuri refugees at Kashuni Camp, Chad, 2005. (Photograph courtesy of Michael Wadleigh/
Gritty.org)*

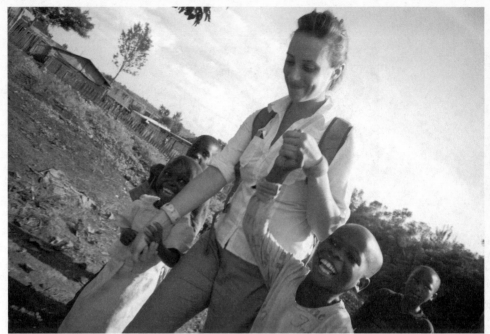

Jocelyn Kelly, Democratic Republic of the Congo, 2009. (Photograph courtesy of Justin Ide/Harvard University)

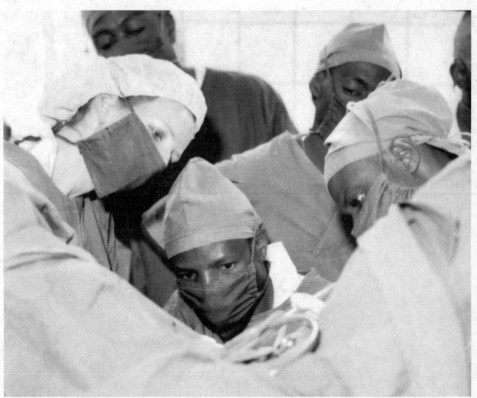

Julie VanRooyen operating at Panzi Hospital, Democratic Republic of the Congo, 2008. (Photograph by the Harvard Humanitarian Initiative)

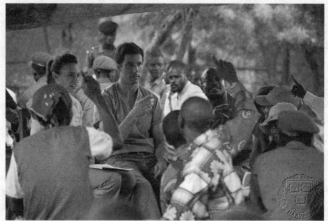

Meeting with Mai Mai soldiers with Jocelyn Kelly, Democratic Republic of the Congo, 2009. (Photograph courtesy of Justin Ide/Harvard University)

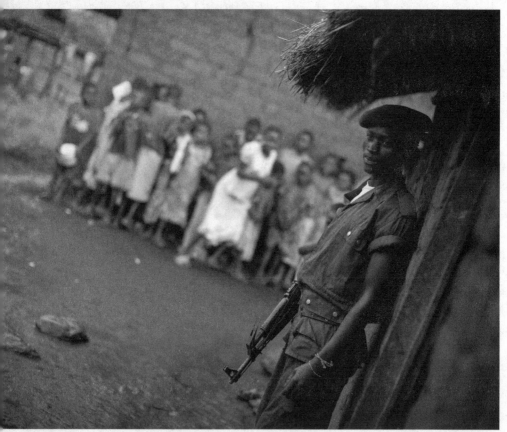

Mai Mai village, Democratic Republic of the Congo, 2009. (Photograph courtesy of Justin Ide/Harvard University)

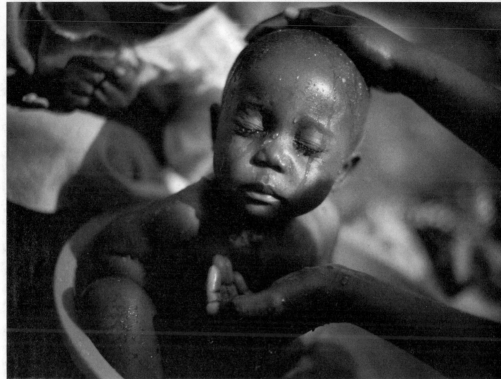

Taking a bath at Panzi Hospital, Democratic Republic of the Congo, 2009. (Photograph courtesy of Justin Ide/Harvard University)

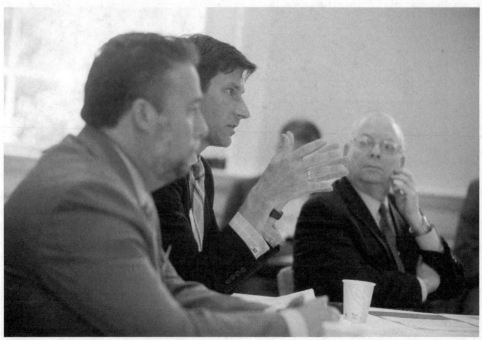

Ambassadors discuss Ebola strategies at Harvard Humanitarian Initiative, 2014. (Photograph courtesy of Harvard University)

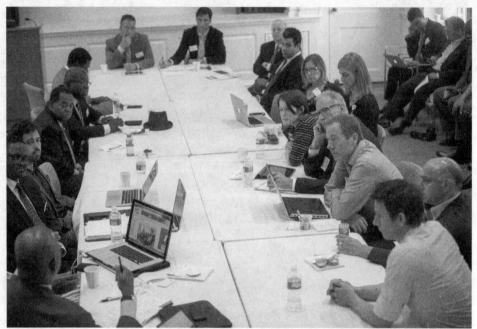

Meeting of ambassadors during Ebola crisis, 2014. (Photograph courtesy of Harvard University)

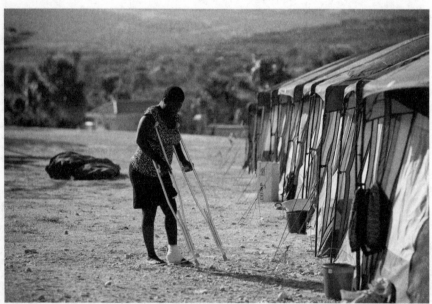

Recovering at the Disaster Recovery Center, Fond Parisien, Haiti, 2010. (Photograph courtesy of Justine Ide/Harvard University)

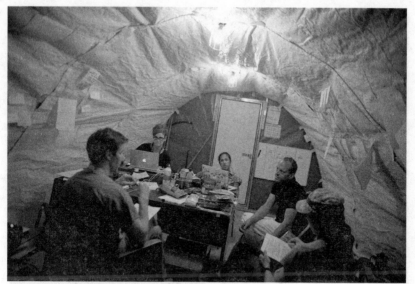

Disaster Recovery Center, Fond Parisien, Haiti, 2010. (Photograph courtesy of Justin Ide/ Harvard University)

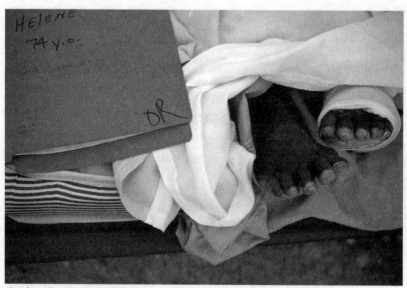

Earthquake survivor, Fond Parisian, Haiti, 2010. (Photograph courtesy of Justin Ide/ Harvard University)

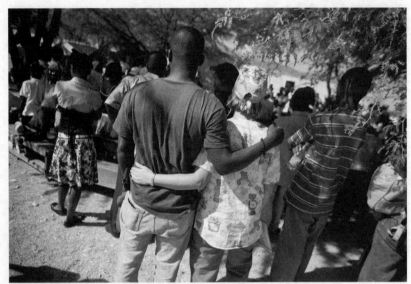

Gathering at the hospital, Fond Parisien, Haiti, 2010. (Photograph courtesy of Justin Ide/ Harvard University)

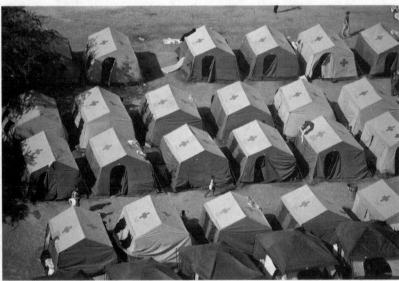

Disaster Recovery Center, Fond Parisien, Haiti, 2010. (Photograph courtesy of Justin Ide/ Harvard University)

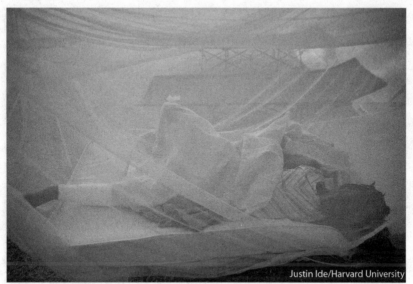

Recovering under mosquito netting, Fond Parisien, Haiti, 2010. (Photograph courtesy of Justin Ide/Harvard University)

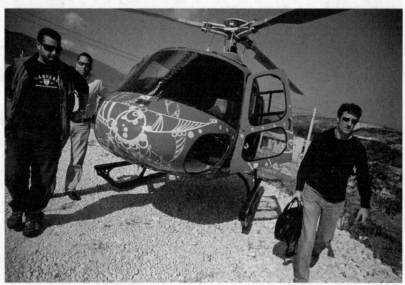

Arriving after the earthquake in Port Au Prince, Haiti 2010. (Photograph courtesy of Justin Ide/Harvard University)

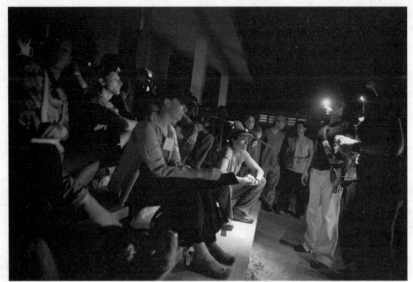

Medical team meeting, Fond Parisien, Haiti 2010. (Photograph courtesy of Justin Ide/ Harvard University)

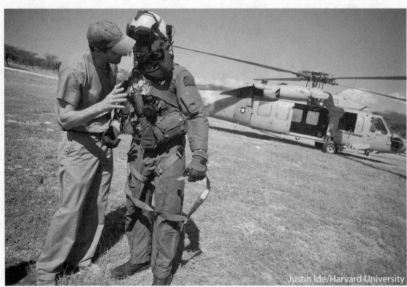

Receiving patients from the USNS Comfort, Fond Parisien, Haiti 2010. (Photograph courtesy of Justin Ide/Harvard University)

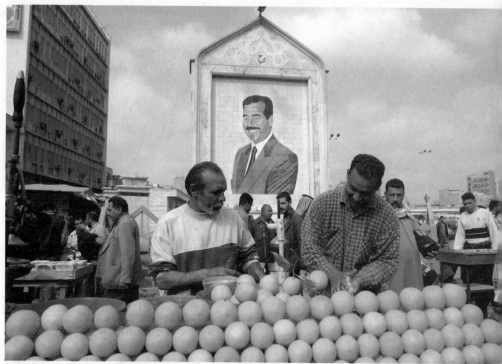

Baghdad market, Iraq 2003. (Photograph courtesy of CESR)

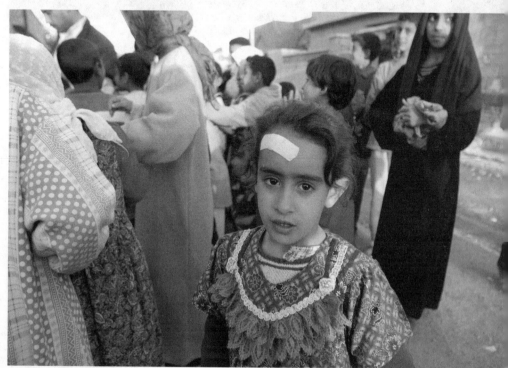

Baghdad, 2003. (Photograph courtesy of CESR)

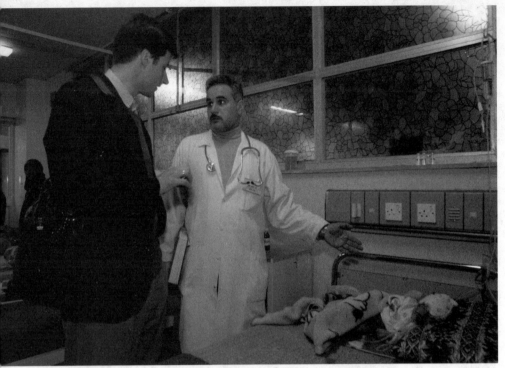

Rounding in Baghdad, 2003. (Photograph courtesy of CESR)

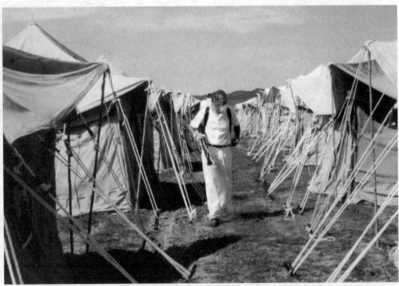

Kosovar refugee camp in Kukes, Albania, 1999. (Photograph by Michael VanRooyen)

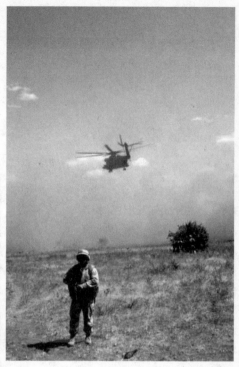

Assessment mission near Baidoa, Somalia, 1993. (Photograph by Michael VanRooyen)

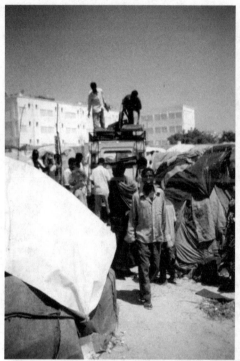

Refugee health program, Mogadishu, Somalia, 1993. (Photograph by Michael VanRooyen)

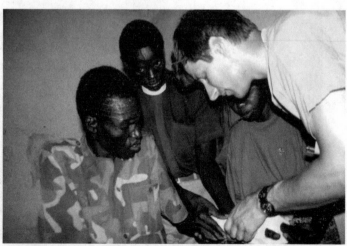

Operating on an SPLA soldier, Maridi, South Sudan, 2000. (Photograph by Michael VanRooyen)

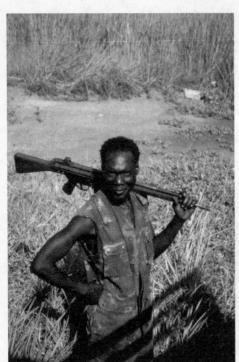

Lui, South Sudan, 2000. (Photograph by Michael VanRooyen)

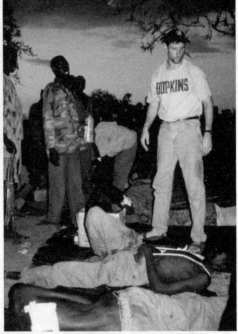

War wounded in Tindalu, South Sudan, 2000. (Photograph by Michael VanRooyen)

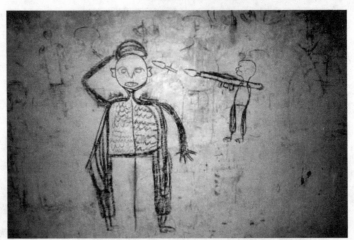

War art at Lui Hospital, South Sudan, 2000. (Photograph by Michael VanRooyen)

6

FINDING
HUMANITARIAN SPACE

THE RUINS OF THE TWIN TOWERS LOOKED LIKE A BI-
zarre movie set. Walking among the twisted metal and concrete skel-
eton of the World Trade Center, I could not imagine that two 110-story
skyscrapers had actually stood there. The colossal pile of rubble was still
burning, filling the air with heat, fumes, and acrid smoke.

I arrived with an emergency medicine colleague at New York's
Ground Zero on September 14, 2001. We had driven from Maryland
to Manhattan, hoping to contribute our emergency medicine expertise
to the search for survivors. We brought our medical gear, dust masks,
and hard hats. After passing through a security checkpoint, we looked
around for makeshift medical clinics that had sprung up around the
wreckage that could use our help.

Firefighters, policemen, and rescue teams in hard hats and masks crawled over burning mountains of rubble, searching for any sign of life. The searchers were covered with gray dust and exhausted from working through the night. They refused to go home. They dug methodically into the heaps, pulling debris away by hand and sending it down along a bucket brigade line. They searched any accessible spaces, hoping against hope to find anyone alive in the wreckage.

One firefighter suddenly whooped. "We've got one alive!"

Other rescuers rushed toward him and joined in the furious digging. An optimistic buzz surrounded their work, and all efforts focused on reaching that side of the pile. But soon the celebration stopped. The firefighter had been mistaken. The diggers delicately pulled out another body from the pile. My colleagues and I stood by, stunned. Amid the chaos, every worker stopped. Helmets came off, and heads bowed as the corpse of another victim was carried away. There was little hope that anyone could have survived under the millions of tons of burning rubble. Nevertheless, the rescuers all returned to "work the pile." The bucket brigade reformed, and the search continued. Along the base of the pile, I could see several bodies covered by heavy rescue tarps. Soon these victims would be somberly carried away by firefighters to a staging area nearby, joining the dead already recovered from the wreckage.

Leaving the pile, we entered what had been the lobby of One Liberty Plaza and was now a temporary morgue. Marble that had gleamed the day before was covered with dust, debris, and emergency workers. Papers, memos, and financial documents littered the area, the remnants of normal business in the days before the attack.

As we passed through the lobby looking for one of the medical treatment units, the building started to shake. Firefighters yelled for everyone to get out, and we ran toward the doorways. I slipped on the wet marble floor and fell hard, striking my right hand on the ground and breaking it. I would not realize it was broken for two weeks. We quickly moved clear of the building, which eventually proved to be stable. The immense pile had likely just been settling, shaking the deep foundation of the World Trade Center site. I found a first aid station, got an ace wrap for my hand, and continued to look for a way to pitch in.

I spent the following week working with the American Red Cross as a volunteer physician-epidemiologist. During that time period, the number of people working increased exponentially, and access to the site was soon tightly controlled by security. Eventually, only workers with official access badges and security clearance were allowed into the area. Scores of medical teams arrived to set up operations, but just a few hours after the attack, it became clear that there were no survivors. All the medical teams could do was treat the minor injuries sustained by the crews that were still searching. The smoking mountain of metal and concrete created a constant feeling of dread. It became clear that Ground Zero was a massive forensic and cleanup effort—a crime scene, not a medical emergency. After several days on site, I finally went home, emotionally drained.

In the days after the attacks, news reports confirmed that the terrorist organization al-Qaeda had orchestrated the events of 9/11. The world changed that day, and we could feel it. The attacks on the World Trade Center, Pentagon, and United Airlines Flight 93 were the deadliest terrorist events on US soil ever, killing 2,996 people and causing over $10 billion in damage. Instantly, 9/11 caused a sea change in modern geopolitics. The international "War on Terror" began, eventually leading to the invasions of Afghanistan and Iraq and expanding the political and cultural gap between the Middle East and much of the Western world. The War on Terror reshaped politics, governments, and millions of lives over the following decade. The fields of international relief and development were no exception.

Since the creation of the first Geneva Conventions of 1864 and the subsequent updated treaties of 1949 in the aftermath of World War II, civilian humanitarian action has rested on a critical principle: aid agencies are independent of governments and impartial in their provision of care. In practical terms, the protection afforded to aid agencies in conflict settings historically has been based on their perceived neutrality. Acceptance by local communities and governments of this neutrality provided a safe and generally secure working environment for humanitarian aid providers that allowed aid agencies to work on both sides of a conflict. But the policy climate in the post-9/11 West changed—in major, irreversible ways—the connections among aid, diplomacy, and politics. These changes profoundly shifted the perception of aid in recipient countries. In this new era, aid was no longer seen as neutral, and agencies providing humanitarian aid in conflict settings were no longer guaranteed security.

First among the changes was the polarization of the globe. Just as the Cold War defined aid efforts in the 1970s and 1980s, the War on Terror branded nearly every international humanitarian action with a geopolitical identity. Aid agencies from the United States and Europe, even those not funded by US governmental grants or contracts, were identified as being on the Western side of the War on Terror. This association was particularly perilous for groups working in Afghanistan and Iraq. NGO and UN personnel in those countries had once enjoyed a degree of recognition of neutrality. In the post-9/11 world, these agencies were increasingly targeted—for harassment, abduction, and, in many cases, murder. The era of "neutral aid" was coming to a close, and organizations were forced to adapt.

Second, the US government made it clear that US-based NGOs receiving government funds were an integral part of the nation's foreign policy. As a result, the perception of these NGOs changed. They were now seen as extensions of the American government, and part of a strategy to improve global public opinion of the United States, rather than simply altruistic humanitarians. The use of aid to engender goodwill is neither new nor novel. But in the aftermath of 9/11, the use of foreign aid as an instrument to improve the public image of the United States and advance US foreign policy placed NGO personnel's lives in danger in a new way. For example, after catastrophic floods in Pakistan in 2010, US-AID required that bags of food distributed there bear a "USAID: FROM THE AMERICAN PEOPLE" stamp. International aid agencies found that such branding placed their staff at grave risk of harassment or attack, and lobbied to have the stamp removed from food deliveries to this region.

An additional complication stemmed from post-9/11 US and European legal policies that expanded the definition of "terrorist organization." These policies also forbade partnering with any group that could possibly be linked to anti-Western activity. This had the practical result of severely restricting local partnerships in areas that US-based organizations could not easily access. Previously, local organizations often formed the backbone of effective relief programs in conflict and post-conflict settings. But after 9/11, many local relief programs on the ground in conflict areas were suspected of having terrorist connections and could no longer function without the assistance of larger international groups. Aid spending became less efficient.

Third, the increasing military support of aid efforts in conflict zones eroded the perception of neutrality. As the provision of humanitarian aid evolved as a central strategy for the Department of Defense, the US military increasingly used aid to win "hearts and minds" in some of the most politically complex areas. The Provincial Reconstruction Teams in Afghanistan exemplified this concept of military–civilian collaboration, bringing together military protection forces and civilian government officials from USAID to promote political stability and begin the process of reconstruction. The logistical muscle of the US military proved useful in delivering aid after natural disasters like the 2010 earthquake in Haiti. But the use of American military assets for humanitarian aid in active combat zones underscored that such assistance is no longer neutral, nor can it be seen as separate from American foreign policy objectives. The blurring of lines between civilian and military efforts meant that all aid came to be viewed as linked to Western foreign policy. While "militarizing" aid was undeniably useful in areas like Afghanistan that were too dangerous for civilian organizations, the collapsed distinction between civilian and military aid deeply undermined the foundation of the humanitarian community. Those aid agencies whose missions were neutral and independent now operated in a world where they were seen as neither.

This change in perception had very tangible results in the field. NGOs with global operations were seen as partners with foreign governments, and their presence in a community was often met with suspicion, if not outright hostility. The traditional founding precepts of humanitarian aid—neutrality, independence, impartiality and humanity—were sidelined. In the new geopolitical reality, no one knew if these guiding principles could ever be completely restored.

This growing threat to the neutrality of aid was, unsurprisingly, most pronounced in the Middle East. As US-led wars and reconstruction efforts in Afghanistan and Iraq revealed a clear plan for nation building across the region, friction on the ground surged. The environment for aid operations in the Middle East was punishingly complex, and nowhere more so than in Israel and the Palestinian territories.

Jerusalem is at the center of many complex and dynamic disputes, with both Israelis and Palestinians identifying the city as their capital. While many accept that Jerusalem is the capital of Israel and East Jerusalem is the capital of the Palestinian territories, Jerusalem is recognized by the United Nations as belonging to neither the Israelis nor the Palestinians. In the eyes of the United Nations, the entire city remains a UN-administered entity, as laid out in the original partition plan approved by the UN General Assembly in 1947. The city and surrounding area, including the city of Bethlehem, are also referred to as the "Holy Basin," and they remain a flashpoint for political, religious, and cultural divisions across the region.

In September 2000, a year before the 9/11 attacks, conservative Israeli prime minister Ariel Sharon paid a controversial visit to the Temple Mount complex in the heart of Jerusalem's Old City. Sharon's visit touched off a series of violent Palestinian protests and Israeli retaliations. The violence escalated into the Al-Aqsa Intifada, or Second Intifada. The exact causes of the conflict are disputed, as with nearly every aspect of Israeli–Palestinian fighting. Some blame Sharon for staging a deliberate provocation, while others accuse the Palestinians of using the visit as a pretext for violence that had been planned well in advance. Regardless of the cause, over the course of the next five years, more than 1,000 Israelis and 3,000 Palestinians were killed. Suicide bombings, abductions, and targeted killings escalated. Security at border crossings tightened. Many of the clashes that took place between Palestinians and Israeli Defense Forces (IDF) soldiers occurred at border checkpoints.

I went to East Jerusalem for the first time in 2002 to work with CARE International on expanding the capacity of emergency health systems there. Experts from Johns Hopkins worked with CARE to develop partnerships with local Palestinian organizations, including the public health authorities and ministries of health in Gaza and the West Bank. The goals of the CARE program were to advance emergency medical capacity and trauma care, and to conduct a number of studies on the medical and public health consequences of the ongoing intifada, including the effects of roadblocks and checkpoints that separated Israeli territory from the Palestinian territory on access to health care. At that time, the UN Office for the Coordination of Humanitarian Affairs reported the existence of 522 roadblocks and checkpoints impeding the movement of Palestinians. The checkpoint system created a de facto ban on travel between certain parts of the Palestinian territories and severely hampered travel between home and work, to markets and schools, and to hospitals and clinics.

When I arrived, the security climate was intensely strained, and access from Israel to Gaza and the West Bank was severely restricted. I traveled with a convoy across the heavily armed checkpoint between Gaza and Israel, heading for Gaza City and eventually the city of Khan Yunis. We were to meet with the Palestinian minister of health in Gaza to discuss a series of educational programs and research studies that we hoped to launch as part of the CARE program. Every checkpoint crossing was tense, and it felt as though fighting could erupt at any moment.

One of the most important and volatile checkpoints was in Qalandia, the main crossing between the northern West Bank and Jerusalem and the site of attacks, protests, detainments, and violence inflicted by both sides. The Qalandia checkpoint was first erected in 2001 after a wave of suicide bombings and was used by the Israeli military to monitor and control traffic between East Jerusalem and the Palestinian city of Ramallah. Every day, hundreds of Palestinians lined up to pass the checkpoint with permits for work, worship, and access to medical services. Ambulances were generally allowed to pass, but only after inspection.

When we arrived at Qalandia, we stood along the heavy concrete barriers in a long line of men, women, and children carrying bags of groceries, all waiting for clearance. The checkpoint was crowded, and the air carried an anxious charge. The hot wind blew sand across the crowded lines, and I turned to shield my eyes from the dust. At a signal from heavily armed soldiers, border crossers approached the cinderblock-and-sandbag station to have their documents inspected and to present their reasons for crossing. While we waited to cross, two men carrying an older woman were trying to get through the line quickly, presumably seeking urgent medical attention. There was some pressured confrontation with the guard, who eventually called another over. After more conversation and an inspection of their bags, the three were allowed through to meet a taxi on the other side.

Although this group was able to accelerate its crossing, long delays in transit across checkpoints were frequent. The Qalandia crossing had seen a number of "checkpoint births" as pregnant Palestinian women went into labor and delivered outside, still in line for inspection. The system of barriers has been blamed for major health and economic problems in the Palestinian territories. In 2011 the *Lancet,* the premier journal for global health affairs, published a controversial series of articles highlighting the health and humanitarian implications of the roadblock system and the ongoing effects of obstructed access.[1]

Standing at Qalandia, the process did feel dehumanizing. I talked to a few Palestinians in the long line, but they were guarded and brief in their replies. We were herded along the fence and pushed more tightly together with nowhere else to go. For the first time since I had arrived, I felt hopeless. I could see just as clearly the effects of the constant threat of terrorist attacks on Israel as I could see the impact of Israeli checkpoints on the daily lives of Palestinians. Qalandia felt like no solution at all.

We spent the next weeks developing a program that would ultimately become a detailed study of the effects of these checkpoints on the Palestinian population. The research program was difficult. Led by my colleague Gregg Greenough, a fellow emergency physician from Hopkins, the study surveyed households affected by the roadblock system. We found that the health consequences of the tight control were far-reaching, including malnutrition and iron deficiency anemia. As the study's results were being analyzed, it became clear that the findings would be an intensely political issue. On August 6, 2002, our conclusions were published in the *Lancet* and were picked up by both scientific and popular media. The study showed that the Israeli-imposed closures contributed to acute malnutrition in one in five young Palestinian children, a rate similar to those in Chad and Bangladesh. It also noted that the Gaza Strip was profoundly affected by the roadblocks, with more than 22 percent of children under the age of five suffering from acute or chronic malnutrition, a level that constituted a humanitarian emergency. In both territories, over half of the Palestinians had restricted access to food.

The responses to this study varied widely. The Israeli restrictions were an obvious target of commentary, but there was also significant criticism of the suicide bombings and terrorist attacks that had led to the imposition of these travel restrictions. The Israeli military took great interest in the results of the study, which were not contested by Israeli health officials, to better grasp the impact of the roadblocks on civilian life, and to find ways of loosening restrictions while maintaining security. Perhaps ironically, of all of the organizations to react to the study, the IDF was the only one to act decisively to improve access.

The onslaught of attention that the study received taught me another lesson: impartial research is powerful. I had entered Gaza and the West Bank with no preconceived opinions about who was right and who was wrong, and our team had aimed to produce a truly unbiased evaluation of the health impacts of the political situation. The data needed to speak for itself. Ultimately the objectivity of the study was the best argument for its validity. The fact that we were scientists from a university using a clear methodology created an important perception of neutrality on an otherwise intensely political issue. The work taught me an important lesson about the power of objective research and the ways such research can be translated into policy change, both affecting larger governmental objectives and assisting the actions of organizations working on site. This research would encourage the IDF to open up borders to increase Palestinians' access to food and medical care, and would create an argument that many areas in Gaza and the West Bank needed supplemental food aid and a lifeline to areas with aid resources.

At this time, field research was beginning to contribute in important ways to the understanding that war has profound, unintended, and deadly effects on civilian populations, far beyond the simple danger of bombs and bullets. Modern conflicts deprive civilians of health care, food, and safety. Noncombatants trapped in conflict areas suffer just as much, if not more, than soldiers on the front lines. The notion of "excess mortality"—the difference between the death rate attributable to a crisis and the normal death rate—was easy for the public to understand. Research highlighting the causes of excess mortality began to impact policy and politics. In fact, the very concept of excess mortality challenged the logic and morality of military intervention, and would become a lightning rod for controversy in the Second Iraq War.

In January 2003, a second US invasion of Iraq seemed imminent. The War on Terror was expanding. US military campaigns in Afghanistan, Pakistan, and the Horn of Africa pursued terrorist organizations like al-Qaeda. Plans for an invasion of Iraq and the overthrow of Saddam Hussein were in the final stages. There was little hope that war could be averted. But in the lead-up to the invasion, there was a growing sentiment among many Americans that conflict should be averted through diplomatic means, and that an invasion would only lead to further regional instability. Furthermore, the invasion was strongly opposed by most of the United States' traditional allies, such as France and Germany. Many felt that additional civilian diplomatic efforts might help tip the balance toward a peaceful solution. When I was asked to join a delegation to Iraq tasked with evaluating the true humanitarian implications of a possible war, I immediately said yes.

The delegation with which I traveled to Baghdad was organized by the Center for Economic and Social Rights (CESR), a human rights organization. Our mission was to quantify the impact of the humanitarian crisis that Iraq would face in the aftermath of the impending invasion. We would collect data, interview representatives from several ethnic groups, and author a report summarizing how war would harm the civilians of Iraq. Our group included Hans von Sponeck, the former assistant secretary-general of the United Nations, who had previously served as the UN humanitarian coordinator for Iraq, overseeing all UN activity in the region, and Ron Waldman, a seminal figure in disaster epidemiology from the CDC and USAID and a pioneer in humanitarian policymaking. Also in the delegation, to my happy surprise, was Charlie Clements, in whose footsteps I had followed in El Salvador more than ten years earlier.

The delegation spent several weeks traveling around the cities of Baghdad, Mosul, and Kirkuk in the north, and Basrah in the south, with the goal of interviewing physicians, businessmen, local politicians, and average Iraqis to get an idea of the potential consequences of war for their country. The health team evaluated twelve national hospitals to understand the impact of sanctions and the future consequences of conflict. I focused on the southern city of Basrah. Basrah was near the Iranian border and had been devastated by the Iran–Iraq War of twenty years earlier. That conflict had lasted for eight years and killed over a million soldiers, many by chemical warfare. By the end of the war in 1988, medical services in Basrah had collapsed. Recovery had been short-lived. When Iraq invaded Kuwait in 1990, postwar sanctions brought the Iraqi economy to its knees and once again decimated hospital services. Physicians again had to work without reliable labs, X-rays, or surgical facilities.

To see if hospitals in Baghdad had suffered the same fate under sanctions, I met with medical staff at the Saddam Pediatric Hospital in Baghdad and asked how they were preparing for the upcoming war. The physicians were demoralized by the decline in their hospital over the last decade, and many of them were angry that international sanctions under the Oil-for-Food Program (OFFP) had cut off their access to critical medical supplies needed to run the hospital. The OFFP, drafted by President Bill Clinton in response to the economic impact of sanctions on Iraqi citizens and ratified by the United Nations, came into effect in 1996 and provided modest relief from sanctions. The program, which aimed to prevent Iraq from building up its military, allowed Iraq to sell oil on the global market in direct exchange for food, medicine, and other humanitarian needs without allowing the transfer of cash. But corruption, waste, and bureaucratic delays essentially froze access to most medical materials. The results were catastrophic. Iraqi doctors who were used to practicing the highest level of medical and surgical care in the region were now powerless to run their hospitals. The Iraqi healthcare system could no longer manage high-end surgical care, cancer care, blood banking, or trauma. The system was crumbling, and they had no resources to prepare for the impending war.

Having grown up in a place where you could freely criticize your local and national leaders, it was hard for me to comprehend the paranoia of physicians who felt that they were constantly under scrutiny, and that saying the wrong thing to the wrong people might get them killed. But this was exactly the impression I got when talking to medical staff in Iraq. They declined to comment publicly on the political implications of the Hussein government. In confidence, many of the physicians I spoke with worried about the political effects of an invasion. Many thought that the destruction of Saddam Hussein's Baathist Party would leave a power vacuum and create new tensions between the Shia and Sunni. These views, as it turned out, were prescient.

While in Iraq, I met with an old colleague, Margaret Hassan. Margaret was an Irish-born aid expert who had lived and worked in Iraq for many years and eventually married an Iraqi engineer, became an Iraqi citizen, and joined CARE to be their country director for Iraq. I had previously met her at a conference where we sat together on a policy working group, and we now met again in her home office near Baghdad to talk about the preparations that she saw Iraqis making for the impending war. She told me she was deeply worried about the already-weakened state of the healthcare system across the country and the deliberate intimidation of physicians and nurses by the Baathist regime. She also worried about the divide between Shia and Sunni.

"This war will unleash every political and sectarian tension in the country," she said over coffee. "Iraq will become a very dangerous place."

Margaret's fears were more than realized. On March 23, 2003, barely a month after that cup of coffee, the war finally arrived. The conflict began with the American invasion of Iraq and subsequent overthrow of the government of Saddam Hussein. The resulting power vacuum destabilized the region. A rash of sectarian violence broke out between Sunni and Shia, along with an insurgency that targeted occupying US troops, UN staff, and aid workers. The conflict was widely viewed by the global public as unjustified, compounding economic and human costs that were already exorbitant. Public opinion polls in the United States showed widespread disapproval of the invasion. More than one think tank opined that the US-led war and occupation stimulated al-Qaeda recruitment, and that the insurgency in Iraq had become a breeding ground for the next generation of terrorists.

In the aftermath of the invasion, the new provisional government of Iraq asked the United Nations for aid in rebuilding a functioning political process and monitoring human rights. The response was the UN Assistance Mission to Iraq, established by a resolution on August 14, 2003. Just five days after the Security Council adopted the resolution, a suicide bomber drove a truck full of explosives into the Canal Hotel, the UN's base of operations in Baghdad. Twenty-two UN staff members were killed, and many more injured. Among the dead was Sergio de Mello, the UN special representative in Iraq, a head of the mission, and a rising star in the United Nations. De Mello had represented the best hopes for a UN-brokered peace in the region. The attack dashed those hopes and led to an explosion of violence. Most of the UN staff in Baghdad were evacuated within a few weeks. The bombing and subsequent UN withdrawal from Iraq had a catastrophic effect on future UN efforts in conflict areas around the world, one that lasts to this day.

As sectarian attacks escalated, medical staff caring for any patients deemed enemies of the insurgency were targeted and killed. NGO staffers were abducted, and more than 150 journalists and aid workers were killed. On October 19, 2004, my colleague Margaret Hassan was kidnapped. She subsequently appeared in a video pleading for the withdrawal of British troops. Iraqis lined up outside of CARE's offices, demonstrating support for her release, but on November 8, she was executed. Margaret Hassan had dedicated her life to improving the lives of Iraqis. The entire humanitarian world mourned her.

Over the next year, continuing attacks on humanitarians, journalists, and diplomats created a deep sense of foreboding in the aid community. Organizations that had supported health care in Iraq withdrew, as did thousands of Iraqi healthcare workers, leading the nation's health system to deteriorate further. A 2004 study by researchers from Johns Hopkins reported that more than 100,000 excess deaths, most of them civilians, had occurred since the beginning of the war.[2] The study demonstrated once again that civilian men, women, and children make up the vast majority of the casualties in modern war.

Alongside these radical changes in the aid world, in January 2003 my family's world also changed radically when my wife Julie was diagnosed with melanoma, a deadly form of skin cancer. She had already battled basal cell skin cancers, which are minimally invasive and generally removable, and her dermatologist had kept a close eye on her. But the diagnosis of melanoma was an entirely different matter. When caught early, the disease is entirely curable, but if the cancer invades the lymph nodes, the prognosis becomes much less hopeful. Survival rates from metastatic melanoma had not improved much since my mother died of the same disease in 1969. This was stunning news for our young family. Just like my mother, Julie was diagnosed in her thirties. The difference was that we seemed to have caught it early and had access to one of the best medical centers in the world for treatment.

Immediately after the diagnosis, Julie's melanoma was excised, and she underwent a chest CT scan. We were relieved to find out that the disease had not spread. Julie would not require chemotherapy or additional surgery. But while the news about the melanoma was good, the CT also revealed a thyroid mass, which turned out to be thyroid cancer. Two primary cancer diagnoses in one month doubled our shock. We spent the next weeks working up the thyroid cancer, which included biopsies, scans, and lab tests. After an initial surgery to remove the thyroid and treatment with radioactive iodine, Julie was found to have residual lymph nodes that required more extensive surgery and lymph node dissection. After an intense few months, it appeared that both the melanoma and the thyroid cancer were successfully treated. Julie was, to our eternal relief, cured, and she has now been healthy for more than ten years.

Julie's cancer diagnoses deeply affected us both. For her, they created a greater urgency to be even more present in the lives of our children, a decision that would ultimately take her away from clinical medicine—managing a dual-doctor family had proven incredibly complicated. For me, they demonstrated the fragility of life and family. It was a clarifying moment. The need to support Julie and be available to my family made it even more obvious that I needed to reduce my field time and forge a career in which I could be at home more. Several colleagues of mine had recently moved in the opposite direction, assuming leadership of NGO and UN humanitarian operations and spending a greater percentage of their time abroad. The strain on their lives and families was significant. Although I was being pulled more and more toward the field, in the end, the decision to travel less was an easy one. Having gone though such an intense life experience, Julie and I were both ready for a change, and we set about contemplating our options.

In 2003 I began to talk with colleagues at Harvard about the possibility of moving my work to Boston. I wanted to create something brand new, from the ground up, at a powerful academic home. The deeper I dove into the humanitarian world, the less I felt I really understood it.

Building a humanitarian center would take me far outside of medicine and into many other fields. War and conflict created problems that involved diverse disciplines such as anthropology, sociology, public health, economics, and international law. Harvard seemed to be a place where new frontiers could be explored and tested. The prospect was incredibly exciting.

Harvard was also the academic home to one of the most powerful emergency medicine programs in the country. Unlike most premier medical schools, Harvard Medical School (HMS) does not have a hospital of its own but instead partners with a number of well-known Boston-area teaching hospitals. One of the largest of these affiliated teaching hospitals is Brigham and Women's Hospital (BWH), known as the Brigham. This hospital has a long and storied tradition of innovation, and its emergency department is a powerhouse. Many of the leaders of the field have trained there, and the department and its faculty are internationally known.

At this time, Ron Walls, the hospital's chairman of emergency medicine, and my former Hopkins colleague Rich Zane asked me to visit Harvard to discuss the emerging field of global humanitarian aid. Another longtime friend and colleague at Harvard, Jennifer Leaning, joined them in the recruitment. A mentor to me for many years and a teacher of humanitarian studies and human rights at Harvard's School of Public Health, Jennifer was keen to explore ways we could collaborate to expand Harvard's footprint in humanitarianism. After a few trips back and forth to Boston, it became clear that this was a tremendous opportunity, and I accepted a position at the Brigham. It was during one of those flights that I began developing the idea of a university center for humanitarian scholars. As the plane left Baltimore, I pulled out my laptop and set about creating a presentation for this new academic venture. It was short; I made only one slide: "Harvard Humanitarian." It was the first step in a long journey to create something quite different at Harvard.

Jennifer, one of the foremost academic experts and critical thinkers in humanitarianism and human rights, soon became my partner in creating a first-of-its-kind academic program in humanitarian assistance. We aimed to build a center of learning that had one foot in the university and one foot in the field, with the power to change how academics and aid work together. We launched the Harvard Humanitarian Initiative (HHI) in 2005, and it quickly grew into a unique, university-wide program. Based in the university and reporting to the president and provost of Harvard, HHI brings together experts and faculty with an unbelievable wealth of knowledge from nearly all of the schools and centers across the university, including the School of Public Health, the Kennedy School of Government, the Harvard Law School, the Harvard Business School, the Harvard Medical School, and many undergraduate departments. Our goal was simple: to partner Harvard experts with field organizations and create innovative approaches to humanitarian aid. The potential of HHI was powerful; but combining aid fieldwork with academic rigor would prove immensely challenging.

The first major challenge was political. In order to launch HHI as an interfaculty initiative at Harvard, the provost required us to gain the support and buy-in of all of the deans and all of the affiliated hospital presidents. The daunting process of gaining these approvals took over a year, but at the end, we had laid the foundations of a multi-institutional program focused on the science of humanitarian aid. HHI would study and improve the applications of data with the aim of preparing the next generations of aid professionals. In essence, we were building the prototype of a "humanitarian university" at Harvard.

We soon saw a clash of cultures between the university and the humanitarian field. Solving this clash was our second big challenge. NGOs and the United Nations move very fast in humanitarian crises, with rapid scale-up into a powerful field presence in complex, dangerous environments and an emphasis on stretching budgets. Universities (and Harvard was no exception) are slower, more expensive, and more risk-averse; classes aren't typically taught in a war zone. HHI would need to work with field organizations in conflict settings, and HHI faculty and staff soon became embedded in complicated contexts in Chad, Congo, Sudan, Somalia, East Timor, and throughout the Middle East. Deploying technical humanitarian experts from Harvard alongside, for example, MSF workers was a complex endeavor. It was easy enough to find the right people for the right positions, and likewise easy to create new ways of doing field research, but it was hard to move money to Harvard or between its institutions, hard to cover administrative costs, and very hard to do it all quickly.

Then there was the matter of getting a job. My work in building HHI was voluntary and did not pay a salary. I needed a position that afforded me the flexibility, creativity, and academic base to pursue the vision of creating HHI. My grounding in emergency medicine was once again the answer. I joined Brigham and Women's Hospital as a senior faculty member. This way I had a home base in an academic emergency department and a stable platform for building this complicated program at Harvard alongside many colleagues who were also poised to step into this unusual new discipline of humanitarian medicine.

We had navigated the first set of challenges. In the coming years, we would tackle the work of building humanitarianism at Harvard. It felt like a unique moment: standing on the edge of a new field, with the opportunity to build something that could change the aid world.

7

A NEW ERA OF CHALLENGES

I WOKE UP WITH THE SUN, WRAPPED UP IN A HALF-dozen itchy wool blankets inside my UN tent. I was in a refugee camp in eastern Chad, just across the border from the Darfur region of western Sudan. The climate in these borderlands is typical desert: intensely hot and dry during the day and near-freezing at night, when the clear black sky pulls away all of the heat of the day. The night had been especially cold, so I stepped into the sun to warm up.

Outside, I scanned the Kashuni refugee camp, wondering where to find some hot water for instant coffee. I also pulled out my father's pipe and packed it with tobacco. Though I don't generally smoke, I bring this old pipe along on trips as a quiet tradition. I toasted him with a few puffs in the desert dawn. Someday, I would tell him about this place.

Even though it was very early, I discovered that most of the camp of 16,000 had already awakened. Kids were out collecting water. Mothers were building small fires and preparing to bake the flatbread eaten at nearly every meal. The day was already off to a busy start. The bustle of the morning was a sharp contrast to the inhospitable landscape. If not for humanitarian aid (in the various forms of food, water, shelter, and protection), the entire population of the camp would likely have perished. The sand-blasted savannah could support very little vegetation, mainly twisted thorn trees that gave little shelter from the desert sun. The Fur (or Darfuris), the tribal people of Darfur, had been forced to flee to this desert no-man's-land. At home in Sudan, they lived simple, subsistence-level lives in a sparse country that was not much more verdant than eastern Chad. But to the Darfuris, that challenging land was home. Darfur was their birthright, handed down over many generations. There, their lives had been intensely interconnected. Families depended on each other to share food, tools, donkeys, and camels. They needed each other to live, let alone prosper, in the forbidding landscape.

As inhospitable as Darfur was, a lengthy civil war for control of the region had smoldered there for more than a decade, since 2003. I was at the Kashuni camp to understand and advocate for its civilian victims. In this conflict, the government of Sudan had recruited the horse-riding Janjaweed militias (*Janjaweed* roughly translates to "devils on horseback" in the local dialect of Arabic) to exterminate the Darfuri tribes. The Janjaweed originated from nomadic Arab herding tribes already in conflict with the native farming tribes over Darfur's limited water and arable land. Backed by the Sudan government, the horsemen slaughtered cattle, burned farmers out of their villages, and drove them into the desert, killing those who remained behind. The refugees at

Kashuni were fortunate; many Darfuris were killed outright. As many as 200,000 non-Arab Darfurian civilians have died during the war. The extensive disruption of civilian life and extreme violence, especially sexual violence against women, drew the attention of international human rights groups and aid organizations to Darfur.

In January 2005, Physicians for Human Rights (PHR) sent a team to investigate whether the violence in Darfur constituted genocide, as defined in the UN Genocide Convention. The team consisted of myself, John Heffernan, and Michael Wadleigh—a particularly unlikely group. John, our team leader, was a career human rights lawyer working for the Holocaust Museum in Washington, DC, with a long résumé of policy and advocacy work. He was intelligent, thoughtful, and, despite his odd refusal to wear a wristwatch, an incredible organizer. Michael was a seventy-ish hippie and the Academy Award–winning director of the 1970 documentary *Woodstock.* Wiry, with long gray hair and an acerbic wit, he was somewhat eccentric, but he was also intrepid and a brilliant photographer. Michael was there to help us document the systematic destruction of the Darfuri way of life. To ascertain whether genocide was occurring, we needed evidence that the violence had destroyed livelihoods and eliminated all means of survival. The actual work consisted of interviewing villagers from various sites in Darfur to understand what exactly had happened to them: What was the manner of the attack? Why did their attackers destroy everything from livestock to farm tools? Did their experience match that of other villages that the Janjaweed had swept through?

John, Michael, and I traveled across eastern Chad and into Darfur, where we saw for ourselves the suffering that the conflict had brought. Entire villages had been burned to the ground, leaving the charred remains of farm animals among the debris. Blackened pots and broken tools were scattered across the site, making it clear that people had fled the Janjaweed in a panic, leaving behind their belongings and cattle. John and I picked our way among the barren remains of what was once a market, while Michael peered into a well that had been deliberately destroyed and filled with the carcasses of dead animals, preventing anyone from ever using it again. The scene of destruction painted a clear picture. This was not a simple attack on a village; it was the total destruction of a settlement designed to prevent any possibility of return.

As we visited several villages and refugee camps, we spoke to dozens of people who had been forced out of their homes and into the desert. They told us about their family members being murdered, their wives being raped, and their entire way of life destroyed. What we saw and heard made a compelling story, with the destruction and displacement of Darfurians constituting a clear violation of international humanitarian law. The pattern of attacks, rapes, killings, and razing of villages was intended to completely eradicate the Darfuri tribes from western Sudan. The violence in Darfur met every relevant official definition of genocide—those of the Geneva Conventions, the International Criminal Court, and the United Nations. Defining the events in Darfur as genocide constituted an important distinction and a call to action, as the UN's Genocide Convention stipulates that where genocide is determined to exist, member states are obliged to intervene.

In September 2004, testifying before the Senate Foreign Relations Committee, Secretary of State Colin Powell called the Darfur conflict a genocide and made a case for sending an international peacekeeping force to the region. In January 2006, the PHR team presented our findings to members of this committee as well as other congressmen and staffers. Our report would add to the growing political pressure on the UN Security Council to authorize the use of force to protect and repatriate Darfur refugees. On February 18, 2006, President George W. Bush called for the number of international troops in Darfur to be doubled from the 7,000 African Union troops that were already on the ground. Later that year, British prime minister Tony Blair wrote an open letter to the members of the European Union calling for a unified response to the crisis. To this day, however, many of the proposed UN actions on Darfur have been blocked by both China and Russia, permanent members of the Security Council with longstanding weapons-for-oil deals with the Khartoum government. China is Sudan's chief diplomatic ally and the largest consumer of Sudanese oil in the world. The Sudanese military is supplied with Chinese-made helicopters, tanks, fighters, bombers, rocket-propelled grenades, and machine guns. This close alignment with China has protected the government of Sudan from the full weight of international sanctions, and the conflict in Darfur lingers on as a "chronic emergency."

The frustrating big picture in Darfur and my work with PHR sparked our efforts at HHI. We needed to use new research to drive political and operational decision making in humanitarian crises. To make a real impact, HHI needed to be far out in the field, in the most controversial areas, doing pioneering work on humanitarian issues and leveraging this work for policy change. Building such a far-reaching field program at an academic center such as Harvard was daunting. HHI needed to be present and relevant in large humanitarian operations, but Harvard was a very traditional academic setting.

To do innovative work, HHI had to accomplish two things that were often at odds with each other. First, we had to be deeply rooted in current humanitarian crises. Second, we needed to be a credible resource for NGOs and the United Nations. The aid world was dominated by large international organizations that were excellent at providing food, water, sanitation, and health care for thousands of people, but these groups often were not well trained at measuring the impact of their work or quantifying the downstream effects of the aid they provided. This was where HHI could be a valuable resource. HHI researchers were highly skilled at field research and thus had the potential to find new ways to measure the impact of aid and provide the feedback that aid organizations needed to improve their programs. Such a role was an important one, but unusual for a traditional university.

This created a conflict at Harvard. Humanitarian field research is inherently dangerous and requires travel to very remote areas. In addition, field studies have not typically been considered pure research, and this type of fieldwork was neither sanctioned nor recognized by the university. Sending faculty and students to work in conflict and disaster settings on less than twenty-four hours' notice was something that the university could not easily accommodate. In order to get into the field rapidly, I exploited my rather unique position. As a full-time emergency physician at the Brigham, my additional work with the university was voluntary and did not require university financial support. Perhaps because of this freedom, I frequently pushed the limits (and patience) of the administrative team at the School of Public Health and developed a reputation for pressuring the system hard to get my team in the field quickly during major emergencies. I often was called to meet with the staff of the Provost's Office who were, to their credit, generally very supportive. I often joked with my own staff that I was once again being called into the "principal's office," when in fact, this group provided the political backing we needed to grow and prosper at Harvard.

This culture clash was exemplified by the problem of cash. Because my team often operated in conflict areas where there were no banks, we did our business in cash, and we had to carry large sums of money in order to pay drivers, interpreters, translators, and researchers. Harvard isn't in the habit of handing out cash advances at short notice, nor was it reasonable to expect students and researchers to raid their bank accounts before going into the field. So I found a practical solution to the problem. I cashed in one of my personal retirement funds and placed $25,000 in new $100 bills in a zippered bag. When members of my staff needed money, they would come to my office, scribble an IOU on a Post-it note, and trade it for the cash they needed. While a bag of hard currency is not the optimal way to fund academic research, it was the most practical way to cover people going into the field on short notice. My moonlighting as a banker was (quite understandably) frowned upon by the university (and my wife), but it was a necessary measure to move money to the field quickly and keep our projects moving forward.

To build our new concept of academic humanitarianism, we had to have the right people. This meant finding the rare person who had deep field experience in conflict and crisis and would be comfortable sleeping in a refugee camp and conducting research before coming right back to teach university courses in disaster management. Such people are a rare breed. One of the great fortunes of my career, however, has been the opportunity to work alongside Jennifer Leaning, who, in the early years, was my co-director at HHI. Together, we were lucky enough to recruit some excellent young physicians who shared our vision. In particular, Hilarie Cranmer, Stephanie Kayden, and Gregg Greenough showed incredible talent in both the field and the classroom. These emergency physicians from the Brigham each possessed a unique set of skills that made them invaluable in the field. They were smart, motivated, and intrepid. They had trained in public health and amassed significant résumés in humanitarian field response. They were levelheaded and flexible, able to leverage both clinical and public health skills in the field. They created a model for the emergency physician–humanitarian worker, one that would evolve to play a larger role in future generations of humanitarian leadership.

This core team also helped HHI build our educational programs and develop the ways we would train the next generations. One flagship course was the Field Humanitarian Simulation. Over the course of several years, HHI developed a complex simulation of humanitarian fieldwork, held every spring at the Harold Parker State Forest in North Andover, Massachusetts. Using a large stretch of woods, trails, and lakes, we built a realistic scenario for an immersive training experience in humanitarian operations in war and disaster settings. The "Sim" tested everything from organizational and negotiation skills to tolerance of the cold and rain. The course became a draw for aid workers, physicians, UN personnel, and students who would form the future of leadership in the humanitarian sector. Through this exercise and other efforts, HHI aimed to create an "army" of aid workers that understood the changing roles of humanitarian workers, the complexity of crisis, and the need to collaborate. Over the next ten years, we would train over a thousand future leaders in humanitarian assistance, the people who would eventually be on the front lines of future deployments in crisis.

Our training model, and the entire model for humanitarian aid, would soon be tested by a new crisis. On the morning of December 26, 2004, an undersea megathrust earthquake in the Indian Ocean led to the most deadly tsunami in recent history. Surges of up to one hundred feet slammed into coastal areas in fourteen countries, killing

230,000 people. Hardest hit was Indonesia, where in Aceh Province over 130,000 people were killed and half a million displaced. Many coastal communities were completely destroyed, with lives and livelihoods washed away in mere minutes.

The tsunami captured the attention of the world and evoked an unprecedented outpouring of concern, action, and financial assistance. Within a few weeks, governments and NGOs raised billions of dollars. Aid agencies scrambled to join the massive response. Before the tsunami, only a few international agencies had had a local presence in Aceh Province. Immediately after the disaster, 300 international NGOs responded, and thousands of aid workers arrived in Aceh, funded by nearly $10 billion from governments and individual donors. Most of the NGO arrivals had never worked in Indonesia, did not speak the language, and knew nothing of the activities of other organizations. Compounded by Indonesia's deep systemic corruption, the resulting aid effort was one of the most wasteful humanitarian responses in history. New NGOs, looking to build their name in a high-profile crisis, failed to coordinate with other agencies. Work was unnecessarily duplicated. The result of the confusion was not only a massive waste of resources, but a growing public distrust of aid and the organizations that provided it.

Just as the Sphere humanitarian standards were born out of the failures of the Rwandan refugee crisis, the aftermath of the East Asian tsunami drove renewed UN efforts to reform the process of coordinating relief. In 2005, the United Nations Office of the Coordination of Humanitarian Affairs (OCHA) underwent a major reorganization. This translated into changes in the funding, leadership, and coordination of UN responses to major crises. As part of the reforms, the UN "Cluster System" was created.

The Cluster System was formed by the Inter-Agency Standing Committee (IASC) to address the problem of widely disorganized humanitarian programming and to prevent the overlapping and/or neglect of aid provision. At the same time, the IASC promoted a new humanitarian reform agenda to raise the bar for collaboration between the United Nations and various NGOs and to empower OCHA to oversee all activities across sectors. In the Cluster System, there is one cluster for each of the most important areas of humanitarian assistance, including health, water and sanitation, food and nutrition, and security. The health cluster, for example, is led by the WHO and includes major organizations working in health, such as the International Medical Corps and the International Rescue Committee, to allow coordination of health activities in the field. Led by a humanitarian coordinator, a deeply experienced humanitarian leader reporting to OCHA headquarters, the Cluster System has been deployed successfully in several settings with experienced NGOs that have worked closely together before. It has increasingly become the preferred method to coordinate activities in active humanitarian emergencies.

In Geneva and New York, I worked with representatives of major NGOs, UN agencies, and a few universities to craft the vision and operating principles of the new Health Cluster. I focused mainly on the processes and resources needed to coordinate health services in large-scale humanitarian crises like the 2004 tsunami. The reform process touched other aspects of the aid world as well, from UN organization to leadership to financing, ultimately creating a nimbler, more coordinated relief architecture. For example, the Central Emergency Response Fund created a new pool of $500 million for rapid relief efforts, ten times larger than the prior emergency fund. The reform process also brought together lead organizations in each sector of health, shelter, water, and others to proactively plan ways to coordinate before the next crisis struck.

As humanitarian reform advanced, HHI expanded our research partnerships with Medicins sans Frontières, Oxfam International, and the United Nations. We aimed to launch several important research and policy initiatives with the potential to change how crises were managed. The overall demands on the aid community were expanding dramatically. Aid no longer meant simply providing food, water, shelter, and medicine, but had expanded to take on larger issues brought about by war and disaster, including protection and security, negotiation of access, and long-term recovery and sustainability. Increasingly, HHI was involved in helping UN agencies and governments plan for humanitarian response. Our work extended into financial policies, coordination mechanisms, international law, and human rights. The problems facing war-affected populations are, by their very nature, immensely complicated. New wars, especially conflicts involving local militias, have created a new breed of challenges. Combatant groups have increasingly become embedded in civilian communities, creating greater threats to women, children, and other vulnerable populations. This greater entanglement between combatants and civilians required new approaches, new policies, and new data.

One example of this was the conflict in the Democratic Republic of the Congo. The African wars of the 1990s demonstrated the catastrophic extent of conflict's toll on civilian populations. The largest of these conflicts was precipitated by the Rwandan genocide, the displacement of millions of Rwandans, and the subsequent overthrow of the government of Zaire, which was renamed the Democratic Republic of the Congo (DRC). The DRC, neither democratic nor a republic, became the epicenter of a war that raged across central Africa, a conflict sometimes referred to as "Africa's World War."

Violence and corruption had plagued the DRC since the former Belgian colony achieved independence in 1960. Since the overthrow of the dictatorial president Mobutu Sese Seko in 1997, warfare involving tribal factions, rebel militias, and Rwandan invaders had ravaged much of the country. The vast mineral resources that could make the DRC Africa's wealthiest nation had only served to fuel the bloodshed as militias battled for spoils buried deep in the mines of the Congo.

On February 6, 2000, the *New York Times* published a front-page article on the conflict in the DRC that gave a detailed account of the genesis of the war but understated the scale of its humanitarian impact. The piece stated an estimated death toll of 100,000 people in the first seventeen months of the conflict.[1] Subsequent articles quoted this figure, which was perpetuated in policy circles. The source of this misinformation was never clear, but aid agencies working in the DRC knew it to be a gross underestimation.

This underreporting of mortality prompted the International Rescue Committee (IRC) to conduct four mortality surveys in the eastern DRC between 2000 and 2004 to evaluate the humanitarian impact of the conflict in the DRC. The first of these studies was probably the most shocking, revealing that an estimated 1.7 million excess deaths had occurred in the eastern DRC in the first two years of the war, more than seventeen times the number reported by the press. By the time the 2004 IRC mortality survey was completed, that number had climbed to an estimated 3.9 million excess deaths, making the war in the Congo the deadliest humanitarian crisis since World War II.

Perhaps the most important contribution of this research was its role in helping the public understand the true human costs of the war. The IRC studies show that the vast majority of deaths related to war in the Congo were not soldiers, but women, children, and other civilians. Fewer than 10 percent of these deaths resulted from violence or direct attack; most were attributable to infectious diseases, malnutrition, and vaccine-preventable illnesses.

One of the most vicious and salient features of this conflict was the widespread sexual violence perpetrated against the women of the eastern DRC. Although the Second Congo War officially ended in 2002, sexual violence actually increased steadily over the next five years as local militias fought for control of illegal mines for gold, silver, and coltan, a metal ore used in electronics such as mobile phones. Militias like the Lord's Resistance Army would seize control of mining villages, extort money or food from locals, and organize campaigns of rape, abduction, and sexual slavery. The phenomenon became epidemic. In some villages, up to 80 percent of women and girls were raped. Estimates of the number of women raped, tortured, and sexually disfigured in the DRC reached into the millions.

The "weaponization" of rape, or its use to control and intimidate populations, in the DRC was unusual not only in its scale, but in its almost-unimaginable brutality. Many survivors sustained internal injuries that left them barren and incontinent. Some were shamed and shunned by their communities because of injuries resulting from sexual violence. It was not unusual for survivors to sleep on a mat outside the family home, having been forced out of the house because they smelled of urine. Little was known about why this epidemic of violence spread so fast, and even less was known about how to stop it. The United Nations labeled the DRC the "epicenter of rape as a weapon of war."

In this brutal new kind of war, a place called Panzi Hospital was on the front lines, and a man named Denis Mukwege was leading the fight against sexual violence. Denis, the founder and surgeon-in-chief of Panzi Hospital in Bukavu, DRC, met my wife Julie at a fistula surgical symposium in New York, and they became fast friends. She began traveling to Bukavu to develop a fistula surgical support program for HHI, bringing in pelvic surgeons to assist the surgical teams at Panzi. I first met Denis a few months later, in the courtyard outside of his office at Panzi. I quickly picked him out of the crowd as he walked through the courtyard. He was a tall, elegant, soft-spoken man. As he moved through throngs of his patients, mostly women, he smiled and paused to talk, leaning down to touch them on the shoulder. A devout Christian, Denis was the son of a Pentecostal minister. Earlier in his life, he would accompany his father on home visits to ill parishioners but felt that he could better serve these poor communities as a physician rather than by following in his father's footsteps as a minister. He decided to become an obstetrician-gynecologist after seeing women arrive at his rural training hospital near death from hemorrhage and other complications of unattended childbirth. After specialty training in France, he returned to Lemera Hospital, about sixty miles from Bukavu, where he worked until Lemera was destroyed in 1996 during the civil war that overthrew Mobuto Sese Seko. Denis was forced to leave, but not before witnessing attackers kill thirty-five female patients in their beds. In an interview with the BBC in 2013, he recounted the founding of Panzi Hospital:

I fled to Bukavu . . . and started a hospital made from tents. I built a maternity ward with an operating theatre. In 1998, everything was destroyed again. So, I started all over again in 1999.

It was that year that our first rape victim was brought into the hospital. After being raped, bullets had been fired into her genitals and thighs.

I thought that was a barbaric act of war, but the real shock came three months later. 45 women came to us with the same story. They were all saying: "People came into my village and raped me, tortured me."

Other women came to us with burns. They said that after they had been raped chemicals had been poured on their genitals.

I started to ask myself what was going on. These weren't just violent acts of war, but part of a strategy. You had situations where multiple people were raped at the same time, publicly—a whole village might be raped during the night. In doing this, they hurt not just the victims but the whole community, which they force to watch.

The result of this strategy is that people are forced to flee their villages, abandon their fields, their resources, everything. It's very effective.[2]

Over the next ten years, Panzi Hospital grew to a 350-bed facility that provided surgical care, job training, and legal assistance for more than 30,000 rape victims. It is the only facility in the region that performs the complex surgical repairs that many of these women need to regain something approaching a normal life. At Denis's invitation, Julie led several HHI teams to conduct training programs for surgeons at Panzi, with specialty surgeons from across the United States coming to work with the team in Bukavu. Our goal was to increase Panzi's surgical capacity and to double the number of surgical repairs performed each year.

As Panzi grew, so did Denis's profile as an advocate for women. He won the UN Human Rights Prize in 2008 and the Clinton Global Citizen Award in 2011, and received his first of three nominations for the Nobel Peace Prize in 2013. He also became increasingly outspoken in his battle against sexual violence and the groups that perpetrate such crimes. In a speech given on September 25, 2012, at the United Nations in New York, he said:

> I do not have the honor, nor the privilege to be here today. My heart is heavy. My honor, it is to be with these courageous women victims of sexual violence, these women who resist, these women who despite all remain standing.
>
> . . . We need action, urgent action, to arrest those responsible for these crimes against humanity and to bring them to justice. Justice is not negotiable. We need your unanimous condemnation of the rebel groups who are responsible for these acts. We also need concrete actions with regard to member states of the United Nations who support these barbarities from near or afar.
>
> We are facing a humanitarian emergency that no longer has room for equivocation. All the ingredients are there to put an end to an unjust war that has used violence against women and rape as a strategy of war. Congolese women have the right to protection just as all the women on this planet.[3]

One month after this brave speech, five armed men entered Denis's home in Bukavu and held his two young adult daughters and their cousin at gunpoint until the doctor returned. In the confrontation that followed, the men killed Denis's security guard, fired at and missed Denis, and then escaped in his car. After the assassination attempt, Denis fled with his family to Belgium and then to the Boston area for a few months. Julie and I invited him, his wife, and their girls to our home for dinner that December. We didn't speak about the attack at the dinner table, but privately he told me he was still shaken by the experience and worried about its impact on his family. The invasion of his home and attack on not only him, but also his family, affected him deeply. As a parent I understood the difference between personal risk and the risk to the lives of one's family. But Denis and his family were committed to his returning to Panzi. When he did so on January 14, 2013—using a plane ticket his patients had raised the money to buy—he was welcomed home as a hero.

After his return, HHI expanded its work with Panzi Hospital by continuing our training programs and expanding our research based at the hospital. As we worked more in the DRC, we sought to understand the sources of the rape epidemic. Surprisingly little was known about the motives of perpetrators. During one visit to the DRC, we took a team under the leadership of Jocelyn Kelly, one of our HHI researchers, on a search for the dark roots of sexual violence in the Congo. Jocelyn's research goal was audacious. She intended to find the perpetrators of the sexual violence that had occurred in remote eastern villages and to interview them. Her questions aimed to uncover specifics on how sexual violence was used to control and intimidate a community, and to understand the biggest question of all: Why?

Researching sexual violence in the Congo was dangerous. There was no security, no UN peacekeeping force, and no assurance of safety.

Nevertheless, Jocelyn, a young female researcher working alone, gained access to some of the most dangerous militia groups in Africa through persistence and patient negotiation. In preparation for this research trip, we met with a commander of the Mai Mai, a local militia led by warlords notorious for their exploitation of rural Congolese communities. We sat with him in a dark café in Bukavu, with his lieutenants standing nearby, and described the study. He nodded, asked several questions, and then agreed to allow us access to the Mai Mai soldiers. We took our research team across South Kivu Province in four-wheel-drive Land Cruisers to a series of remote villages that were only accessible by dirt roads and rutted paths. Many of these settlements had been pillaged by the militias. These were sites where women had been killed, abducted, or forced into sexual slavery. Our plan was to gather the men who had occupied these villages, discuss the work we were doing, and interview them.

We arrived in one village to find a few militiamen in a clearing. Soon, several dozen men emerged from the bush. They wore shredded uniforms and leopard skins and clutched spears, machetes, and AK-47s. It was an intimidating sight. But Jocelyn and her team were undaunted. They spoke to the militiamen in French, explaining the interview process. Jocelyn stood in the center of a crowd of soldiers, smoking a cigarette and discussing the plan for the day. We would conduct group interviews about overall life as a "soldier," and then individual interviews would dig deeper into these individuals' activities in the civilian community, finally getting to the matter of sexual violence.

I spoke for some time with the commander of the small regiment. He seemed quite candid, so I finally asked him why he was allowing us to interview his men. He told me that "many of these men have done terrible things, but you must understand also that life is very hard for them in this war. I told the men to tell you the truth, because you are not from the United Nations or from an NGO. You are doing research, and that research might help us." I was struck by the clarity of this remark and felt a greater sense of responsibility about the research itself. This was not being done to create a publication for a line on a résumé. This research was needed in order to change policy that would improve the lives of the people and communities of the Congo.

This unusual degree of access has allowed Jocelyn's Women in War program at HHI to pursue an unusual and creative line of research. Her work has continued to push the limits of our understanding of the effects of the war in the region and has become increasingly edgy, exploring the experiences of child soldiers and sex workers and the economies of illegal mining communities. Jocelyn has created practical approaches for on-the-ground efforts by organizations such as fostering greater involvement by both women and men to destigmatize sexual violence and fight a growing rape culture. She has also pushed the policy community of the United Nations for greater attention to the specific protection needs of women. The World Bank, USAID, and several donors have adapted their funding priorities for the DRC based on her work.

Through programs like Women in War, HHI continued to grow and integrate its work into humanitarian practice and policy. We hosted a series of "Humanitarian Summits" that brought together leading academic thinkers from around the world with leaders from major UN agencies and NGOs. Our goal was to help translate the important research being done into improved policies and practices by field organizations. HHI became a center where experts could convene to explore and debate the most pressing issues facing the aid community and emerge with thoughtful solutions. The research we conducted in Palestine, the DRC, and other conflict zones around the world was just the first step in changing humanitarian policy to lead to better, more effective programs. It was gratifying to see our emerging role in the humanitarian community. Each new crisis would create new and complex problems that would require creative solutions. But as has always been the case with modern humanitarian engagement, the challenges would not be predictable. This would again become evident in 2010, when the global humanitarian network would be stretched beyond its limits.

8

PROTECTING HUMANITARIAN MEDICINE

FROM THE HELICOPTER, PORT-AU-PRINCE WAS A PAN-
orama of destruction as far as the eye could see. Three weeks prior, at
4:53 p.m. local time on January 12, 2010, a magnitude 7.0 earthquake
struck the heart of Haiti. Nearly every structure in the capital was affected. Many multi-story buildings simply collapsed vertically, floor
upon floor, into stacks of concrete. Hundreds of thousands of residences
and office buildings were destroyed or severely damaged, including the
National Palace (the official residence of Haiti's president) and the Pal-
ais Législatif, home to Haiti's National Assembly. The earthquake killed
230,000 people; another 200,000 suffered severe traumatic injuries.

Haiti's health system collapsed as well, leaving a shattered country with almost no medical capacity for treating the injured and dying.

In the first days after the disaster, Haitians dug through the rubble by hand in a search for survivors or the bodies of loved ones. Thousands slept in the streets of Port-au-Prince or in small makeshift shelters as many weakened buildings still threatened to collapse. In total, more than 2 million Haitians were displaced internally.

Over the following days, thousands of aid providers would arrive from NGOs, international militaries, churches, and community groups, most with very little experience in a massive crisis. As days stretched into weeks, the influx of NGOs and relief teams would continue as more countries responded to appeals for humanitarian aid. Within a few months, over 1,000 international organizations were providing some form of humanitarian assistance in Haiti.

Now, I flew over the ruined city in a helicopter with the minister of the interior of the neighboring Dominican Republic and Alejandro Baez, an emergency physician colleague from the Brigham. We surveyed the catastrophic damage to Port-au-Prince before heading to meet with the president of Haiti, René Préval, and some of the surviving members of the Haitian leadership (a number of top officials had died in the collapse of governmental buildings) at their temporary headquarters at Toussaint L'Ouverture International Airport, which was also the staging area for hundreds of incoming aid agencies, all scrambling to set up operations. The meeting—an intense, high-pressure one—focused on plans to stabilize Haiti and begin a long recovery.

Compounding the crowded humanitarian situation in Port-au-Prince was the baseline dysfunction of Haiti itself. Chronic poverty, political instability, and a dependence on international aid complicated the aid response and clouded the prospects for a long-term recovery. The city of Port-au-Prince is an overpopulated mass of hastily built, concrete-block dwellings with no urban plan, no building codes, and few discernable land rights. Rapid urban migration had created a crowded, sprawling metropolis with widespread poverty and unemployment rates above 40 percent. Dysfunction was the norm *before* the earthquake hit.

A United Nations peacekeeping force (the UN Stabilization Mission in Haiti, or MINUSAH) had been in Haiti since 2004 to support political stability in the fragile, aid-dependent nation. Even before the 2010 earthquake, Haiti had been repeatedly battered by disasters, both manmade and natural. In 2004, I traveled there to work in the city of Gonaives after devastating rains inundated the north of the country, a region that is almost completely deforested, the land stripped clear by the harvesting of wood for charcoal. Torrential rain had washed down the denuded hills and caused massive mudslides and flooding that killed more than 2,400 people and displaced tens of thousands. The flooding exacerbated political tensions in the region. Given the country's existing problems, the devastation wrought by the 2010 earthquake was predictable. The humanitarian response to the earthquake was, in many ways, just as predictable.

The response represented both the best and the worst of the aid world. The collapse of Haiti's weakened health system created an urgent need for medical and surgical aid. Given the earthquake's location in an urban capital with a functional international airport less than two hours away from Miami, and the round-the-clock news coverage of the vast devastation that began almost immediately, every aid agency, every surgical team, and everyone with a connection to Haiti flocked to

Port-au-Prince. With no governmental control and no oversight, these organizations could, and did, do whatever they chose. Within a few days, hundreds of new organizations had arrived, set up shop, and were performing medical procedures in a frenzy of relief efforts. Thousands of surgeries, including amputations and orthopedic surgeries, were performed in tents and makeshift operating rooms with little light, little anesthesia, and little in the way of recovery space for post-operative patients. The arrival of thousands of unprepared disaster responders led directly to inappropriate and wasteful aid efforts on a large scale. It also created an impossible scenario for coordination.

After the earthquake hit Haiti, the Cluster System was activated. Agencies arriving to work in various response sectors such as health, food security, emergency shelter, and water and sanitation gathered in Port-au-Prince to begin coordinating activities within their cluster. But the Cluster System was not designed to manage the rapid arrival of hundreds of organizations, most of them with little experience and no idea how to interact within this new architecture. Health Cluster meetings suddenly had several hundred participants, and coordination became nearly impossible. The decimated Haitian government was unable to regulate the influx of aid workers, and the UN coordination system could not manage all of these independent responders. Duplication and critical gaps in coverage emerged, and many needs went unaddressed, such as poor housing and inadequate sanitation. This eventually led to a cholera epidemic that claimed the lives of an additional 8,231 Haitians. After a comprehensive review of the responses to the Haiti earthquake and the 2010 Pakistan floods, the United Nations would undertake a further revision of the humanitarian coordination system, an undertaking known as the "Transformative Agenda."

It is important to acknowledge that many lives were saved by numerous professional aid organizations in Haiti. Countless experts came to organize and manage the rapid scale-up of humanitarian aid. The response of many experienced organizations, military teams, and especially medical personnel made a crucial difference for thousands of injured and displaced Haitians. NGOs like Partners in Health, which had twenty years of experience in Haiti, stepped forward to lead the aid effort and continue to do transformative work in rebuilding medical care in Haiti. Valid criticisms of the NGO response, and the waste and corruption that would later come to light, should not diminish our appreciation for the work of the many dedicated humanitarians who stepped up in Haiti and the bravery and fortitude of the Haitian people.

I experienced one such example of professionalism in the aftermath of the disaster. After the earthquake, Alejandro Baez reached out to HHI faculty members Hilarie Cranmer and Stephanie Kayden at the request of the Dominican government, asking for their help with the rapidly growing problem of finding room for injured patients to heal. Within a day, Hilarie and Stephanie had flown to Port-au-Prince. Both were emergency physicians with deep field experience in humanitarian crises. The scene when they landed was already chaotic, with rescue and medical surgical teams arriving hourly and vying for a place to set up their aid efforts. After a search, the HHI team settled on the Love-a-Child Orphanage compound, located in the small town of Fond Parisien, about an hour's drive from Port-au-Prince near the border with the Dominican Republic, and set out to build a medical-surgical hospital where injured Haitians could recuperate. This HHI facility, eventually named the Disaster Recovery Center, filled a massive gap in the humanitarian response in Haiti: the need for rehabilitation.

The center was a joint effort of HHI, the Brigham, and a number of academic medical centers. This temporary field hospital, launched within forty-eight hours of the disaster, would soon become one of the main receiving points for patients from the U.S. Navy hospital ship USNS *Comfort,* anchored in Port-au-Prince's harbor. Helicopters from the *Comfort* flew post-surgical patients to the hospital, which grew into a 350-bed facility that was staffed by hundreds of volunteers from thirteen countries. More than 2,200 patients, recovering from serious injuries like amputations, fractures, and major head trauma, received care from an army of volunteer physicians, nurses, and Haitian medical and support staff at the center.

Walking through the field hospital felt to me like one of our teaching simulations come to life. In staffing the facility, HHI called upon its network of faculty, fellows, and students, both current and former. I arrived to find dozens of colleagues working at the center, treating patients and organizing every aspect of the field hospital. Compounding their contribution was the fact that every tent, every stretcher, and every bit of surgical equipment had been acquired immediately, and for free. The staff worked around the clock, setting up a homegrown electronic medical records system, inventory management, and even an iPhone app that helped track unaccompanied children and verify any adults who took custody of them. In a situation in which child trafficking was an epidemic, we never lost a child.

The feeling of pride I had in Haiti came not from my own work, but from seeing the dedication and ingenuity of so many of my trainees. Hilarie and Stephanie created a humanitarian ecosystem that drew from our former students and collaborators from around the world. The facility itself held a feeling of hope and optimism. In the middle of this extraordinary tragedy was a tent hospital, set out in crisp, right-angled rows, providing first-world medical care. It was neat, clean, quiet, and staffed by health workers who had both a deep knowledge of the humanitarian system and a very personal connection to each survivor. As I walked through the compound, I could watch a physical therapist helping a new amputee get out of bed for the first time, a group of foreign and Haitian staff bringing food to each patient, a nurse changing a dressing on a surgical wound, and a group of physicians and nurses making morning rounds.

The hospital created a cocoon of support and care for some of the most badly injured Haitians and helped them find their way back home. On May 5, 2010, nearly four months after the earthquake, the HHI Disaster Recovery Center discharged its final patients and transitioned into a small clinic for the nearby displacement camp run by the American Refugee Committee. Renamed Klinik Lespwa (Haitian Creole for "Clinic of Hope"), it continued to care for survivors and their families for many months.

Personally, Haiti left me with very mixed emotions. Watching the humanitarian free-for-all unfold provided unwelcome evidence that the aid "industry" had not moved very far beyond the problems of the 1990s. The aid effort in Haiti was overrun by neophytes with good (and bad) intentions that reflected terribly on the entire aid community. My career had been built on the notion that we could professionalize humanitarian aid responses. But the onslaught of novice agencies, inexperienced surgical teams, and disaster tourists created what seemed to be an overwhelming problem that no amount of training or organization could change.

At the same time, some parts of the response gave me hope. It was enormously gratifying to see what Hilarie, Stephanie, and the trained humanitarians at the Disaster Recovery Center had been able to accomplish. I was amazed, and, I admit, relieved, to see the translation of training into on-the-ground field work. In many ways, the HHI-run hospital at Fond Parisien validated that what we were trying to accomplish—training future humanitarians—could work. Haiti demonstrated the need for professionalization in aid. People trained in humanitarian standards, rights-based care, and field medicine, who understood and supported the humanitarian coordination architecture, helped make our program in Haiti work and exemplified what an aid organization could and should be.

It was also encouraging to see how emergency physicians had stepped forward in the crisis response. The growth and maturation of the field of emergency medicine, and the growing footprint of emergency physicians as leaders in the aid world, supported a new pathway for medical leadership in humanitarian settings. Emergency physicians were becoming the leaders and medical directors of the new aid era, often leading health relief efforts by major NGOs. The ability to adapt to an uncertain medical environment, to understand the larger demands on a medical system, and to improvise effectively comprised a skill set that clinicians in emergency medicine could leverage in a powerful way.

When I left Haiti, there were still decades of recovery work and reconstruction left to be done. In the years since 2010, there have been a number of reports criticizing the aid community's lack of efficiency, use of funds, and ability to get results. The successes and failures of the humanitarian response in Haiti convinced me even more of the need to further professionalize the field of humanitarianism. Some of the most successful efforts there by medical and public health experts had illustrated the difference that a professional humanitarian education can make in the field. This new generation of humanitarians understood aid priorities and the importance of applied international norms and standards. As seen in the Fond Parisien hospital, these young humanitarians displayed a unique skill set that transformed their efforts and those of their organizations.

But to truly professionalize the aid world, we needed a humanitarian university, not just an initiative. By this time, HHI faculty had developed and taught several courses in humanitarian studies. Humanitarian education at Harvard was growing in profile and popularity, and HHI had trained over a thousand aid workers from all over the world. But as humanitarianism became more complex, training for its various roles was needed at every level, from undergraduate and masters students to seasoned professionals. To fill this major gap, we undertook a new effort to formalize humanitarian education and expand our reach to professionals in the field. In 2012, HHI launched the Humanitarian Academy at Harvard. It is the first multidisciplinary academic humanitarian training academy in the world, targeting each level of humanitarian education. As the demand for training expanded, the Humanitarian Academy grew rapidly to offer courses and online training, creating a vital community of professionals and educators in humanitarian aid. It also helped build the all-important pathway to professionalization.

As I expanded the work of HHI, the pressures of running a self-funded organization grew. HHI as an organization operated on what those in academia call "soft money." Our entire budget, eventually several million USD per year, came entirely from grants and gifts. When HHI was founded, Harvard provided start-up funding for three years. After the economic downturn, those funds disappeared. HHI and the new Humanitarian Academy would have to survive entirely on smaller grants and gifts. This model was both a blessing and a curse. On one hand, it was the most insecure way possible to run an office. Each of our staff was affixed to one or more grants, which provided the only source of funding for our work abroad. When a grant ended, the employment ended, which kept us locked in a constant cycle of developing new proposals. On the other hand, it toughened our team, ensuring our faculty and staff were creative, self-motivated, and truly understood the aid world. Our office became much more innovative, developing novel ideas and new approaches. In an era when many other similar interfaculty programs ceased to exist, HHI thrived.

We were incredibly fortunate to secure the funding we needed to explore new and untested approaches. Most of our programs were in areas that were not yet mainstream and therefore lacked well-established grant opportunities. The idea of the Humanitarian Academy was exciting, but without our version of "venture capital," the Academy could never have been launched. We were once again fortunate. In 2012, a family friend, Kristin Mugford, introduced me to Jonathan and Jeannie Lavine, two prominent, albeit understated, members of the philanthropic community. I met with Jonathan and Jeannie in the offices of Bain Capital in downtown Boston and shared my vision for the Humanitarian Academy. The connection was instant. Within about forty-five minutes, the Lavines had donated nearly twenty times what I was requesting. I was stunned and, I admit, a little surprised by their interest. As it turned out, they also felt that if we were going to move this complex aid world forward, we needed to build a deeper bench of leaders. Over the years, I have come to develop a close relationship with Jonathan and Jeannie as friends and advisors. Their early investment, and those of many others, not only stimulated new and innovative programs like the Humanitarian

Academy, but also validated HHI within the traditional Harvard community and granted a sense of permanence to our operations.

My employment as an emergency physician at the Brigham played its own important role in securing the future of HHI. As a vice chairman in the Department of Emergency Medicine, I was able to maintain my clinical schedule, undertake major administrative roles in the hospital, and have the freedom to volunteer my academic time to Harvard. Several of the BWH emergency medicine faculty pursued similar arrangements, maintaining a clinical (and financial) base at BWH while teaching courses, conducting research, or heading out to the field with HHI. This network of humanitarian doctors could volunteer this time only if they had a way to support themselves as emergency physicians. Without the backing of the emergency medicine leadership at the Brigham, HHI would have perished.

The model for propelling HHI forward came with a number of challenges. We all had to balance our busy clinical schedules with our work in the field. Frequently, one or more of our emergency medicine physicians would be called to the field on extremely short notice. They would then frantically trade clinical shifts to free up their schedule for work in Sudan, Pakistan, or Haiti. We were fortunate to have a large staff of supportive physicians who were truly committed to helping their colleagues get into the field. As HHI's connections to NGOs and UN agencies increased, our work in the field grew, as did the demands on our network, fellows, students, and staff. Nearly all of our emergency medicine faculty, most of whom had no connection to HHI or the aid world, stepped forward to help support their colleagues in the field.

Meanwhile, those of us working in the field faced increasing challenges to our safety and security. After 9/11, Western aid agencies faced greater pressure from donors to distribute aid from the United States to improve the nation's image. Increased security threats in some aid theaters meant that agencies had less access to needy populations. Aid agencies consequently experienced the phenomenon of "shrinking humanitarian space," or the notion that aid providers were less able to work freely in a number of regions because of direct security threats and safety concerns. These organizations had to get creative, working with local agencies and partners, in order to get access to and operate safely in politically complex environments. This was particularly the case in the Middle East, where the effects of the War on Terror posed greater security challenges for Western aid agencies. The use of humanitarian programs by the US military as a part of reconstruction and stability operations contributed to the perception that humanitarian aid from the West was aligned with American military interests. Programs that distributed food, medicine, and other aid were increasingly viewed as ideological allies of Western governments. Several specific incidents fueled such suspicions and led to major setbacks for humanitarian programs.

A prominent example occurred during the lead-up to the assassination of Osama bin Laden. The CIA had hired a Pakistani surgeon named Shakil Afridi to go from house to house in Abbottabad, Pakistan, under the guise of vaccinating children. The agency instructed Afridi to draw back a little blood in each syringe during the vaccinations so that the DNA of those individuals who were immunized could be analyzed to identify the relatives of Bin Laden. It is not clear whether this strategy worked, and it is thought that Afridi's team was refused entry to the Bin Laden compound. Nonetheless, in a *60 Minutes* interview, U.S. defense secretary Leon Panetta, who had overseen the Bin Laden mission during his time as CIA director, said that the sham vaccination campaign was helpful in finding the al-Qaeda leader. In the aftermath of Bin Laden's death, Pakistani authorities charged Afridi with treason and sentenced him to thirty-three years in prison. His sentence was later overturned, but the damage was done. With the disclosure that CIA covert operations included sham public health workers, immunization campaigns became suspect among Islamic militants, and actual immunization workers came under attack.

Because of Afridi's conviction, the international aid agency Save the Children was expelled from Pakistan, curtailing a health and immunization program that had been operating there for over thirty years. Since 2012, more than sixty polio immunization workers have been murdered in Pakistan, and the United Nations has suspended its polio eradication efforts in that country, where every year 150,000 children die of vaccine-preventable illnesses. The decades-long global polio campaign, funded by the US government and the Bill and Melinda Gates Foundation, had brought the world to the threshold of polio eradication. But now polio cases have increased in three countries plagued by conflict and insecurity: Afghanistan, Nigeria, and Pakistan. In January 2013, Harvard joined eleven other schools of public health in signing a letter urging President Obama to cease the covert use of medical care to gather intelligence. The letter highlighted how this breach in global public trust undermined the very foundations of medical neutrality.

The erosion of neutrality and the shrinking of the humanitarian space offered a glimpse of the future of humanitarianism. HHI and its partner aid organizations have been forced to face the reality that the old world of humanitarian action is disappearing, replaced by new actors and new ways of working in complex settings. There seem to be fewer "safe" areas for aid workers in an increasingly polarized world.

And nowhere in the world poses a more complex—and dangerous—problem for humanitarians than Syria.

The conflict in Syria is so convoluted that it warrants a brief explanation. Since 2000, the government of President Bashar al-Assad has refused to address human rights violations and implement greater social freedoms. In 2011, the Arab Spring movement sparked protests in Syria against al-Assad's dictatorial rule. In April of that year, the Syrian military, using tanks and heavy weaponry, fired on peaceful anti-government demonstrators. The protests soon became a full-scale armed rebellion, eventually leading to the formation of the Free Syria Army, a major threat to Syrian central authority. But the entry of other factions, extremists, and jihadists fractured the opposition, pushing the conflict into a stalemate. The emergence of the Islamic State of Iraq and Syria (ISIS) has further divided the country. ISIS, which grew out of al-Qaeda in Iraq, capitalized on the regional chaos to occupy huge areas of northern and eastern Syria. The entire conflict has been characterized by indiscriminate attacks on civilians, the bombing of heavily populated areas, mass displacement, sexual violence, and the use of chemical weapons. The Syria crisis is now in its fifth year, and a political solution seems further away than ever.

The conflict has created the most complex humanitarian aid problems of our time, being designated a "Level 3 emergency" by the UN Office for the Coordination of Humanitarian Affairs, the highest designation of complexity for an aid operation. Over 220,000 people have been killed and more than 1 million injured since 2010. The crisis has displaced 7.6 million Syrians within the country, and almost 4 million more are refugees in neighboring countries. It has decimated the economy, the education system, and the security of the nation, and created an entire generation of unemployed, uneducated Syrians with few prospects for the future.

Health care in Syria has also collapsed. In the five years of conflict, over half of Syria's hospitals have been badly damaged or destroyed, and attacks on medical facilities have escalated, forcing the abandonment of many hospitals and clinics. Airstrikes on medical clinics and aid convoys have become commonplace, and many medical facilities now operate underground. Hospitals will not display the organizational logos of their international partners for fear of reprisal. To compound this problem, only a fraction of the country's trained medical staff remains within its borders. In January 2014, Physicians for Human Rights estimated that 15,000 Syrian doctors had fled the country. In the besieged city of Aleppo, only 250 physicians, just 4 percent of the prewar total of 6,000 doctors, remained. This collapse of the medical system has come at the time of greatest need. Syrian citizens cannot travel across lines of conflict to access health care. Performing surgeries is nearly impossible, medications are severely restricted, and public health has collapsed, as evidenced by the first polio outbreak in Syria in fifteen years.

An unusual feature of the war in Syria has been the complete loss of medical neutrality. The conflict has been especially notable for its vicious attacks on physicians, nurses, ambulances, and hospitals, as well as the obstruction of access to health care for sick and injured patients. The bombing of dense urban settings combined with deliberate attacks on civilians create an impossible scenario for rescuing injured noncombatants. Those wounded in urban bombings cannot be extracted from the rubble or evacuated to hospitals because of the risk of direct attacks on first responders—in the forms of ambushes, sniper attacks, booby traps, and unexploded ordnance.

The Geneva Convention of 1864 created an international under-standing that hospitals, ambulances, and medical staffs of opposing militaries are neutral and must be protected from direct attack dur-ing armed conflict. These accords were updated in 1949 and 1977 to address the complex civilian concerns raised by new types of conflict and threats. The Geneva Conventions have long been a fundamental tenet of international humanitarian law and a bulwark of protection for civilians, noncombatants, and medical workers in war zones. Various parties in the Syrian regional conflict have not only ignored these core conventions, but have specifically targeted medical personnel and used the deprivation of health care as a weapon of war. Over 400 doctors, nurses, and medics have been killed in the conflict, and many more de-tained and tortured. Most of these attacks have occurred in retaliation for treating members of the opposing side.

Andrew Bostrom, an HHI researcher, interviewed healthcare pro-viders in and around Syria to explore the reasons behind the deliberate targeting of the medical community. Bostrom's report for Physicians for Human Rights, entitled *Human Rights Violations in the Syrian Health System: Perceptions, Beliefs, and Attitudes about Justice and Accountability,* describes attacks on health care and direct threats to medical neu-trality in exacting detail. In one interview, a pharmacist who had fled from Idlib Province noted: "We were afraid. We were afraid that we would die because of this. They killed doctors; plucked out their eye-balls and pulled out their fingernails. Every kind of torture, just because the doctor was . . . a humanitarian. He was trying to treat, to help a hu-man, a brother of his nation, a brother of his country." Another health worker who had fled to Turkey spoke frankly of deliberate violence against physicians: "There was shelling of field hospitals, liquidation of doctors working to treat the revolutionaries. They were arrested and killed, or sometimes forced to work with the regime to save the lives of [their fighters]. The regime tried to determine the locations of the hospitals and shell them without regard for the presence of people who were inside the hospitals, whether they were civilians or military."[1]

Some of the traditional protections of aid workers have failed to provide immunity in Syria. The Red Crescent emblem—the Arab world's Red Cross—no longer deters attackers. At least twenty Syrian Arab Red Crescent volunteers have been murdered in Syria while treating the wounded or delivering relief supplies.

The attacks in Syria stand out in a global landscape of increasing threats to healthcare workers. In 2013, the International Committee of the Red Cross released a report entitled *Violent Incidents Affecting Health Care,* which documented 921 violent incidents against medical workers during armed conflict and other emergencies in twenty-two countries during the 2012 calendar year alone.[2] These attacks included killings, kidnappings, threats, and denials of passage, and have increasingly targeted ambulances, first responders, and vaccination workers. State security forces are most often the perpetrators of these assaults.

Recognizing this global erosion of medical neutrality, the US Congress introduced the Medical Neutrality Protection Act of 2013. This legislation reiterated that medical neutrality is "an integral part of the defense of recognized international human rights law and international humanitarian law." The Act required denial of American foreign aid to nations that have violated medical neutrality, and also would have incentivized foreign governments to protect health and healthcare workers. Unfortunately, the House of Representatives has no power to improve the situation in Syria, where there is little respect for humanitarian norms and no accountability for attacks on hospitals and physicians.

The work of the entire humanitarian community in Syria, including that of HHI, has been hindered by security and access challenges. We have been able to send a number of our staff to work with NGOs and UN agencies in the region, but a greater on-the-ground presence is restricted because of safety concerns. Furthermore, the expansion of ISIS-controlled territory threatens to cut off access to even more regions. Even in those places to which HHI analysts, researchers, and technical experts can get access, their "space" for work is limited.

Yet the aid community has adapted considerably to find new ways of working in Syria. Despite the difficult security circumstances, in the last two years, OCHA and the UN High Commission for Refugees have created a complex, multi-country structure, including Lebanon, Jordan, and Turkey, to provide corridors of aid into Syria and surrounding countries. Recently, the Whole of Syria (WoS) Cluster Coordination Group also has been formed to coordinate all cross-border aid activities. This innovative coordination scheme is the most complex in OCHA's history, and the rapidly changing political and military climate presents the greatest coordination challenge ever seen by the aid world.

In May 2015, Will Cragin, one of my students, graduated with his Masters of Public Health degree from the Harvard School of Public Health with a concentration in humanitarian studies. Will came to the school already quite experienced and worked with HHI in the field in the Congo and Ukraine while still in class. He was part of HHI's new approach to humanitarian education, with its focus on both theory and field skills. As his mentor, I was very pleased to know that he had landed a high-level field position as the health cluster co-lead in the Syrian response. Will's job is as important as it is difficult, as he is working to coordinate the health sector response in the most complex relief operation that exists today.

I e-mailed Will shortly after his deployment to the field to learn more about his new position in Syria and his experiences there so far. I was also curious about the extent to which his education and training at HHI had prepared him for this job. After my experience with humanitarian practitioners in Haiti, I was convinced of the value of humanitarian training, but was not sure how it would translate to work in the complex response setting of Syria.

Will described his work in Syria as complicated by the physical barriers of hundreds of checkpoints and the political barriers of the UN system. In the absence of a true political solution and ceasefire, the humanitarian system has been called upon to provide aid in a highly charged security environment. The clusters were now increasingly led by NGOs, who were able to successfully negotiate regular access into Damascus, Syria's capital. He noted that he felt as prepared as any twenty-eight-year-old could be for the responsibility of leading the cluster, and that his training with me had helped.

Will also highlighted another crucial requirement for success in the field: emotional intelligence. The secrecy and siloed nature of the various response organizations has led to a pervasive lack of trust, even among aid agencies. Given that trust was probably the most important tool that Will had to gain access and coordinate the complex health programs involved in the Syrian response, one of the most significant contributions he could make was to break down those barriers and create an environment of trust. His experience reinforces the fact that in order to work with many types of actors and in a complicated political environment, developing trust is an essential element of gaining cooperation. Learning to move fluently between stakeholders in the field requires a combination of field experience, in-depth understanding of the political context, and a sense of emotional intelligence.

As I corresponded with Will, I came away with several other important themes. Although Syria is undoubtedly a complex and difficult environment for humanitarians, many aspects of the relief system are working. Despite all of the mistrust of Western intervention, aid workers are being given increasing levels of access within Syria, even as a political solution remains elusive. The implementation of the Cluster System in Syria, while extremely complicated, appears to have been successful. Changes made to the humanitarian coordination system after the Haiti experience have led to a new generation of clusters. Led primarily by NGOs and guided by the United Nations, these clusters have greater flexibility to coordinate efforts in crises such as those in Syria.

The experiences of Will, Andrew, and many of my other students and colleagues working in the field also underscore the complexity and intensity of the humanitarian environment in Syria. As the most destructive and far-reaching humanitarian crisis of the decade, the Syrian conflict has shaken the very foundations of humanitarian assistance. Aid is no longer seen as independent of government influence, nor is it always perceived as neutral. In the future we will face an aid environment that is more dangerous, more constrained, yet more crucial than ever before. This attrition of neutrality means that foreign aid workers will continue to be obstructed and targeted. Sectarian threats like those we have seen in Syria and ISIS-controlled Iraq will expand, and resistance to foreign intervention will likely increase. The original nineteenth-century architects of international humanitarianism could not have imagined that aid workers would be systematically killed for their trade, or that aid would be used for political purposes to undermine peace and security.

In addition, future aid recipients will be far more informed, and aid agencies will need to adapt to the information age. The era of humanitarians passing out food in organized refugee camps to grateful, uninformed recipients is nearing an end. Future aid providers must leverage communications and networking in a more connected and information-rich world and develop better tools to determine who needs aid and how to deliver that aid efficiently, with a view toward longer-term sustainability. At the highest levels, the coordination mechanisms that we have in place must evolve as well. The primacy of international bodies like the United Nations will be further challenged as aid agencies exert their own independence. The field of humanitarian aid will continue to diversify, with foreign governments, militaries, and private industry taking a bigger role in relief and reconstruction efforts.

In the complicated, often-cloudy future of humanitarian aid, one reality is clear. The need for emergency humanitarian assistance will grow. Regional conflicts are expected to spread and morph into new crises, further dispersing populations that will require emergency assistance. The number and severity of natural disasters will escalate, fueled by the compounding effects of rapid urbanization, climate change, and weather extremes. These crises will disproportionately affect the most vulnerable populations on the globe and will require faster, larger, and more sustained relief efforts.

As natural and manmade disasters increase, there will be a greater demand for professional responders who understand how to work in this dynamic and often-dangerous field. Aid agencies will continue to negotiate with armed actors and to establish diplomatic relationships to protect and serve civilians where governments and normal diplomatic channels have failed. If humanitarians are going to evolve to manage the ever-changing nature of conflicts and crises, adaptation is key. The humanitarian approach to Syria shows that the aid world is willing and can evolve to address crises as they arise. As future conflicts and disasters emerge, these same aid agencies will need to contend with new challenges, new actors, and new approaches to serving the most at-risk populations in the world.

9

DESIGNING THE FUTURE OF HUMANITARIAN MEDICINE

A CONVOY OF NORTHERN SUDANESE TANKS, TRUCKS, and artillery units rolled across the rutted dirt roads, heading for the Abyei region. A border district with a population of 20,000, Abyei had become the latest flashpoint in the conflict between the government of Sudan in the North and the world's newest sovereign nation, South Sudan. Just weeks before, on July 9, 2011, a national referendum supported by the vast majority of Southern Sudanese people had declared independence for South Sudan. It was well understood that the separation of South Sudan from the North would leave several of Sudan's most valuable oil fields in the hands of the new nation. Consequently, it was expected that the Northern government in Khartoum would attempt to attack and destroy several towns and villages in the South in order to reclaim this oil-rich territory. This expectation was now a reality, and the government of Sudan's army was pushing closer to Abyei.

At the same time, 450 miles up in the thermosphere, a satellite operated by a company called Digital Globe was taking a series of high-resolution, high-definition images of the border between North and South Sudan, including the Abyei region. The images—massive amounts of data measured in terabytes—were then transmitted at regular intervals to servers in Cambridge, Massachusetts.

At 1:00 a.m. on a Thursday night, the streets of Cambridge and Harvard's campus were quiet and dark. But on the second floor of HHI, all the lights were on, and the office was buzzing with activity. The Satellite Sentinel team was crammed into a conference room, surrounded by pizza boxes and monitors. As the digital images came down from the satellite, the team could watch, almost in real time, the troops and vehicles massing for an attack on a city 6,000 miles and seven time zones away. They were working on an analysis of the satellite imagery from the night before, which was due to be delivered to our partners.

Nathaniel "Natty" Raymond, a veteran human rights researcher with experience in both policy and field investigation, led the Satellite Sentinel team. We had first been introduced by my close colleague Charlie Clements in a small office at the Harvard Kennedy School. Natty's name belied both his appearance and his personality: glasses askew, unruly hair, and a wild gleam in his eye. When Natty started talking, he owned the room. During our first meeting, he gestured wildly to animate his description of an idea that was, well, wild.

"You want to do what?" I asked him, looking around at the others in the room to see if anyone else thought the idea was crazy.

"Use satellites to do human rights investigations in Sudan," he repeated. "It's never been done before."

"Really? How are you going to get satellite data?" I asked.

"George Clooney," Natty replied matter-of-factly.

He explained that one of the major barriers for collecting reliable humanitarian or human rights information in remote areas like Abyei was the lack of any type of data. Without sending a team in to work on the ground, which was costly and dangerous, there was no way to use traditional data collection methods to gather information and no way to know what was going on. There was therefore no way to verify threats to civilian villages in the Sudanese borderlands without seeing the Northern troops move in and position themselves to strike.

Clooney, a Hollywood star and human rights advocate, along with John Prendergast, a well-known *New York Times* reporter, had been working to prevent escalation of the conflict between the governments of North Sudan and the newly minted nation of South Sudan. Clooney and Prendergast conceived the Satellite Sentinel Project (SSP) after an October 2010 visit to South Sudan. They suspected that once the South formally seceded from the North, the Khartoum government would attempt to seize the oil-rich territories lost in the split. Through the use of satellite imagery, SSP could create an early warning system to detect military movement, provide crucial data to responders, and potentially deter mass atrocities by focusing the world's attention on the attackers.

Clooney and Prendergast's approach was outwardly simple: obtain high-quality imaging from the commercial satellite provider Digital Globe, partner with HHI experts to analyze the data, and corroborate the information using ground reports to create an accurate real-time understanding of the threats unfolding in South Sudan. Natty Raymond assembled and trained the team of analysts, and in December 2010, the SSP program came online.

Over the course of the next weeks and months, SSP would explore the power of satellites as a means to hold the government of Sudan accountable for invading a sovereign nation and attacking civilian populations. The use of satellite imagery for humanitarian purposes was brand new. There was no rulebook or "typing guide," the term used to describe the process of interpreting satellite imagery and matching it with known types of buildings, vehicles, or weapons. Satellite intelligence work belonged almost exclusively to military or government intelligence agencies. In a sense, even the instruction manual for this type of work was classified. While some imagery was available to humanitarian agencies, there were no guidelines for reliably identifying military or civilian facilities. As a result, the field lacked both a professional set of ethics and technical standards. Anyone collecting and analyzing data needed a process to verify and authenticate what they were seeing. Natty and his team took on the task of writing the rulebook, using reporting standards employed by the *New York Times* to corroborate findings in the field with at least two independent sources of information.

Largely, however, SSP's analysts learned on the job. The team produced twenty-eight reports and analyses of the new war between North and South Sudan. Their work described what the satellites were seeing: a rapid buildup of troops and munitions, the razing of villages, and the displacement and killing of civilians. The satellite imagery even provided grim evidence of mass graves by detecting the emission of a methane plume produced by the decomposition of bodies below the ground. SSP became one of the only academic programs in the world specifically dedicated to developing the approach and ground rules for accurate, professional, and evidence-based use of satellite technologies in working with vulnerable populations.

As the reports were delivered to Clooney's organization, the profile of the program escalated rapidly. Clooney presented SSP reports produced by HHI to President Obama in the Oval Office—and that was just the beginning. Speeches in Congress and the House of Lords showcased SSP and its work. Testimony at the International Criminal Court cited the program, and more than 10,000 media stories brought SSP to the world's attention.

As the Satellite Sentinel Program grew, it was renamed the Signal Program on Human Security and Technology. The name change reflected a shift in focus: the new signal program looked more toward developing general ways that digital satellite imagery could be used. What was once a rarely deployed tool by UN or government experts at the headquarters level has become a growing part of the humanitarian toolkit. Advances in the amount of commercially accessible satellite imagery, as well as the spread of technologies such as Google Earth, have allowed humanitarian agencies to effectively use visual data in the field to determine concentrations of refugees, map access routes for aid, and survey areas damaged in disasters.

Technological advances in the humanitarian aid world in communications, mapping, networking, and information management are all what I call "humanitarian technologies." These technologies have enhanced how we gather, share, and use information in real time and can drive the management of field programs. The availability of secure but seamless data-sharing platforms means that organizations can enhance their coordination by sharing information such as the locations of communities that need aid and names of organizations working in a particular area. However, the explosion of new tools unfortunately has been difficult for organizations to track. Crowdsourcing data and mapping tools can help reach humanitarian aims, but verifying the accuracy of these sources brings another set of challenges. Likewise, the use of humanitarian drones has become commonplace but has also created significant controversy. Private drones were widely used in Nepal after the 2015 earthquake and raised significant privacy concerns from that country's government. Moreover, the drone work in Nepal did not result in data that helped to coordinate the response. As we have seen from many recent large-scale responses, usable solutions for effective coordination have proved elusive. The control of information by the United Nations may create a more secure system, but many local agencies working in the field still utilize unsecured, easily accessible platforms, like Facebook and Twitter, to share information, organize their work, and track aid recipients. This information can be used in areas of conflict to intercept aid and even threaten recipients. Aid efforts are still routinely undermined by poor collaboration between competing agencies, and new technologies have yet to make fluent, real-time, on-the-ground information sharing an everyday reality.

Imagine you are part of an advance team from a major international NGO and have arrived in Manila just after 2013's Typhoon Haiyan, a Category 5 superstorm, has ripped through the central Philippines, leveling several major population centers. Much of the archipelago is without power, communications, or access to basic needs like emergency water, food, and shelter. You and your colleagues arrange for transportation, meet with local officials, and do a "quick and dirty" assessment of what types of aid are needed. Because your NGO delivers health services, you focus on health, immunizations, and essential medications. Based on surveys, you develop your program, hire your team, and provide initial services like mobile clinics and emergency measles vaccinations.

Now imagine that forty new NGOs arrive and do the same thing—that is, they send a team to do an assessment, collect their own information, and develop a delivery plan. The government has not even started collecting data, and the UN office has yet to provide any numbers on the size and scope of the affected population. All of these assessments and surveys done by the NGOs stay in the hands of each individual NGO. Unless the aid groups collect data in the same way, on the same platform, the information that drives their programs can never be merged, shared, or used to coordinate services. It is effectively lost.

This lack of on-the-spot sharing of information is not only common, but the norm. As a result, organizations have no ability to learn from each other on the ground in real time. The opportunity to coordinate is lost almost immediately. Dozens of organizations work alongside each other, but they can't provide their information to each other, to local providers, or to the ministry of health. This pattern of aid agencies rushing to the field to gather their own information for their own programs creates a cycle of *un*-coordination and *non*-collaboration. This disconnect creates waste, duplication of services, and competition among agencies for the same funds for the same work. It also puts a strain on local populations, the very people who have recently experienced a devastating disaster. Survivors, often reeling from the loss of friends, family, and belongings, hear the same potentially traumatizing questions over and over, seemingly for no purpose. Easy-to-access areas are flooded with aid, while more remote areas want for crucial assistance. Even as professional relief agencies understand the need to coordinate and work hard to optimize their efforts through the Cluster System and other efforts previously discussed, the crisis of coordination persists. We need to determine how data can be used to enhance coordination rather than undermine it.

The power of shared data can be illustrated through another look at our hypothetical response to Typhoon Haiyan. Imagine your organization has worked with the United Nations to adopt an open-source standardized data collection system that is free for all organizations to use. This system allows you to ask standard questions about the medical care, medications, and immunizations given to members of communities displaced by the typhoon. After you gather information from several communities, you upload your data to the cloud, where it is immediately combined with the data gathered by several other agencies working on health issues and analyzed. Within a few hours, you can see a map of communities, providers, and needs. Such a system shares the critical knowledge collected by each participating NGO—and powers a new degree of coordination and efficiency in relieving urgent humanitarian needs.

In 2010, Patrick Vinck and Phuong Pham, a husband-and-wife research team at the University of California, Berkeley, moved to Harvard to develop a new software solution for sharing information in an aid crisis. Their KoBo Toolbox has now been tested in more than thirty countries and adopted by OCHA to systematize the collection and sharing of data across organizations. Now one of the most widely used data collection systems in humanitarian crisis response, with over 5,000 active users, KoBo Toolbox adds to the coordination potential of the Cluster System, enabling it to work as designed. In March 2014, Eric Schmidt, Google's executive chairman, recognized the importance of the KoBo Toolbox approach by bestowing one of the company's "New Digital Age" grants on HHI to support a new expansion of the KoBo software. The support of Schmidt, the United Nations, and several other donors allowed KoBo to expand into new frontiers of information collection and management. As data systems like KoBo grow in popularity and become normal operational practices for NGOs and UN agencies, hopes for more coordinated crisis responses are beginning to feel realistic.

Data sharing, mapping, and remote imagery have given aid agencies new tools to enhance their response and accountability, but work remains to be done. New global policies and new ways of incentivizing collaboration among competing agencies must also be developed. The 2004 tsunami in Southeast Asia, the 2010 earthquake in Haiti, and the ongoing Syrian crisis have shown us that the aid community will always have to adjust to the changing nature of crisis. This reality is illustrated by the recent West African Ebola crisis, which created yet another serious challenge to the prospect of turning humanitarianism into a true profession.

In March 2014, I received a call from Ken Isaacs, my longtime friend and the head of international programs for Samaritan's Purse. After working in Liberia for more than a decade, the organization had taken over an MSF-run Ebola treatment facility in Liberia. The Samaritan's Purse staff had closely trained with MSF. With more than 300 international workers and 3,000 national staff, MSF was the largest agency working in West Africa and had set the global standards for Ebola treatment, infection control, and epidemic containment. After a month of managing the Ebola treatment center, Ken told me that the growing Ebola epidemic was unlike anything he had ever seen before. Both Samaritan's Purse and MSF were struggling to get the World Health Organization and the CDC to recognize this new Ebola outbreak as a public health emergency with global implications.

The Ebola outbreak that began to spread in late 2013 was thought to originate from bats living in caves in central Africa. Humans who ate those bats and other game meat were infected, and Ebola then rapidly spread to other humans through contact with blood, sweat, and saliva. The virus was deadly, killing nearly half of those people infected. As an Ebola case progressed, vital organs would fail, and the delirious patient would bleed from the eyes, nose, and mouth, spreading the virus to the doctors, nurses, and caregivers who were working to save them.

Prior Ebola epidemics had been contained in small rural villages. Like many diseases, Ebola preyed on the poor, and its spread was abetted by weak health systems and poor health education. The 2014 epidemic was different from previous outbreaks, in part because of geography. This time Ebola flared up at the intersection of three countries: Liberia, Sierra Leone, and Guinea. People who had been in contact with an Ebola patient traveled back to their respective villages and cities, and the epidemic rapidly spread to the urban centers of all three nations.

On July 26, Ken Isaacs called me again. Samaritan's Purse physician Kent Brantly had just tested positive for Ebola. The doctor had developed a fever after working in the organization's Ebola Treatment Center in Monrovia and became the first American aid worker infected by the virus. Shortly afterward, nurse assistant Nancy Writebol, who had worked alongside Brantley, also tested positive. In light of these events, Ken Isaacs needed a plan for the quarantine of dozens of Samaritan's Purse staff members who may have had the same exposure. We discussed evacuation plans and which US facilities would be prepared to accept Ebola patients. This problem was so new that there were no protocols and no practices in place. The CDC had not created clear guidelines for Ebola response, and the WHO had declined to identify Ebola as a public health emergency. Ultimately, Ken arranged to have Brantly and Writebol flown to the United States in a modified Gulfstream III aircraft equipped with a unique biological containment system. Brantly and Writebol were transported to Emory University Hospital, one of four hospitals in the United States with the capacity for managing Ebola patients, and were the first people to be treated with the experimental drug ZMapp. Though initially critically ill, both survived and recovered.

As the threat of an explosive epidemic that crossed international borders became very real, MSF and Samaritan's Purse struggled to raise critical awareness. The treatment of Brantly, Writebol, and other Ebola patients, and several subsequently infected Western health workers— including an American doctor named Craig Spencer, who tested positive for Ebola after arriving home in New York after working for MSF in Guinea—created a significant public panic. Suddenly US hospitals were scrambling to prepare for the possibility of an exposed patient showing up in their emergency departments. Finally, on August 8, 2014, the WHO's International Health Regulation Committee declared the Ebola outbreak a global public health emergency. Ministers of health, ambassadors, and other world leaders gathered in the United States to discuss their national strategies for preparedness and response.

Shortly after the WHO announcement, Jim Yong Kim, the president of the World Bank, asked me to come to Washington, DC, to meet with global leaders at the organization's headquarters to examine the global strategic response to Ebola. Jim, a former colleague at Harvard, is a physician-anthropologist and the co-founder of the Boston-based NGO Partners in Health, in addition to his leadership position at the World Bank. He had led HIV/AIDS programming for the WHO before coming to Harvard and was well aware of the implications of a global pandemic. I arrived at the meeting to find the table full of the world's leading experts in health and epidemic management, including Tom Frieden, director of the CDC; Tony Fauci, director of the National Institute for Allergy and Infectious Disease; and Margaret Chan, director general of the WHO.

The message from Jim was clear. The WHO response had been slow, the US response was too internally focused, and we needed aggressive action to enhance every aspect of the Ebola response. We needed more doctors and healthcare workers, more experienced organizations, and more public health programming to screen and educate the public. There were several major barriers to controlling the epidemic, and we needed a roadmap for getting around or through them. One major hurdle was that Ebola created a unique and difficult problem for traditional responders. Ebola-infected patients require intensive medical care and extremely strict infection control. There was little local capacity in West Africa to achieve these levels of patient safety, and many health workers had already died taking care of Ebola patients. The complexity of the medical care and infection control, and the extreme risk to healthcare providers prevented most organizations from stepping in to assist. Running an Ebola treatment center was no task for a novice organization, and even an NGO with health sector experience likely did not have the advance funds and technical medical capacity to build a treatment center, intensively train staff, ensure a pipeline of medical supplies and protective equipment, and provide the assurance that any infected staff would be evacuated immediately. Even when the aid community fully mobilized, very few agencies were able to provide Ebola treatment services. We needed a reliable influx of personnel with specific expertise and a complex support system to ensure that they could function safely.

Ebola had decimated West Africa's already-weak health systems, including the medical staffs of its major hospitals. Prior to the outbreak, Liberia had about 50 doctors for the entire country of 4.3 million people, or roughly one doctor for every 100,000 people. The United States, by contrast, has 250 doctors per 100,000 people. Brigham and Women's in Boston has 1,200 physicians on staff—more than 20 times the number of doctors in all of pre-Ebola Liberia.

One of the most important programs that emerged in Liberia was developed by Michelle Niescierenko, a pediatric emergency physician and HHI fellow who directed global health efforts for Boston Children's Hospital. She had worked in Liberia for several years prior to the epidemic, training new physicians in the country's teaching hospitals. As she watched the epidemic overrun Liberia's hospitals, she saw large sectors of the healthcare system close down because of lack of staff, lack of protective gear, and lack of physicians. The public hospitals in Liberia became dangerous for both patients and staff, sending health care in Liberia into deep crisis.

Determined to support the cadre of young physicians she had trained, Michelle, with the assistance of Kayla Enriquez, another HHI fellow and BWH emergency physician, launched a program called AC-CEL (the Academic Consortium Combating Ebola in Liberia) that would support the few remaining doctors in Liberia as they stepped forward at the most crucial moments of the epidemic. As others were abandoning Liberia's government hospitals, she created four Ebola infection control training teams and sent them to train and equip all of Liberia's twenty-one government hospitals. Aided greatly by Michelle's investment into preparing these medical leaders, Liberia's hospitals began to recover. While many Ebola-related aid efforts shut down after the worst of the crisis passed, ACCEL has continued to grow.

In the United States and in Boston we struggled with the simple process of getting our physicians to work in the Ebola epidemic. The public paranoia over the return of a few infected patients to the United States created a high-profile preoccupation with domestic safety and a general aversion to sending our healthcare workers abroad. Fears of both danger to the individual provider and a subsequent exposure of the hospital system loomed. Several of my colleagues from hospitals outside of Boston had already headed to the field to work with NGOs that were building medical capacity in Liberia and Sierra Leone. Before we were allowed to send anyone to the field from the Brigham, we had to verify, beyond doubt, that the NGOs running these Ebola treatment centers had the capacity to keep our physicians and nurses safe, and to safely evacuate them if they contracted the virus.

The skepticism was understandable. With public paranoia over Ebola growing, it was difficult to convince the Boston hospitals that we should send our physicians into battle. Finally, after many committee meetings and many refusals, the emergency department at the Brigham was the first in our healthcare system to directly fight the epidemic. We ultimately sent two physicians to Sierra Leone to work with Partners in Health (PIH), a Boston-based NGO that had a long history of deploying Brigham physicians. Regan Marsh and Shawn D'Andrea, both emergency physicians experienced in international missions, cleared their clinical schedules and mobilized to the field to help build the PIH Ebola treatment facility. They knew the risks, as much as anyone who deploys into the unknown can, but I spent several sleepless nights worrying about sending them to West Africa. They worked for the next two months to jumpstart the new PIH Ebola program in Port Loko, Sierra Leone. The risk they faced was very real. A month after their return, two healthcare workers from the same facility, one American and one from Sierra Leone, contracted Ebola. The infected American was evacuated to the National Institutes of Health bio-containment unit in Bethesda, Maryland, and the patient from Sierra Leone was treated in the Ebola treatment center in Freetown, Liberia's capital. Both eventually recovered, much to our relief. But the close call hit home with PIH and many in the NGO world.

The Ebola epidemic brought a new and unexpected dimension to crisis response planning that was different from that seen in other recent crises. The earthquake in Haiti, for example, had all the elements of a perfect storm: extreme severity, high publicity, and easy accessibility, encouraging responders of any type to mobilize and begin work without direction or control. In contrast, the Ebola epidemic led to a slow response and delayed NGO engagement in the disaster. The combination of a remote geographical location with a deadly and unpredictable disease made even the most experienced aid organizations hesitant to enter the field. NGOs had to reckon with a threat to their own staff that could also follow them home to affect their domestic population. Many professional aid agencies found themselves unprepared for and intimidated by the prospects of tackling the threat of a growing pandemic. Only a few stepped forward.

The Ebola crisis also occurred within the context of the ongoing humanitarian needs of the wider world. As the West African emergency was evolving, the UN and the humanitarian community were also deeply engaged in different crisis settings around the globe. The United Nations defines the highest-intensity humanitarian crises as Level 3 emergencies. As the Ebola crisis peaked, it competed for aid resources with an unprecedented four other Level 3 humanitarian crises in Iraq, South Sudan, Syria, and the Central African Republic—the largest number of simultaneous Level 3 crises since the 1990s. Each aid theater required the deployment of the full UN humanitarian coordination system. Simultaneously, the aid world was struggling to address the needs of an estimated 51 million refugees and internally displaced persons, the highest number of displaced individuals since World War II. The Ebola epidemic arrived at a moment of intense strain on the finances and manpower of international NGOs and UN agencies.

These forces have all contributed to a humanitarian aid environment that is dynamic and sometimes unpredictable. Much of my current and future work with HHI involves anticipating the drivers of change in the aid world. Predicting the needs of the humanitarian community for the next ten, or even twenty, years is a complicated calculus that includes geopolitical trends, patterns in climate migration that drive populations to urban centers, and the types of resources that will be required by the next generation of humanitarians. Any plan for effective aid responses will have to confront a new set of working conditions and unforeseen complications.

Developing and growing a professional workforce remains an issue of crucial importance. Over the past decade we have often struggled to improve the professional path for future humanitarian leaders, even as the need for those leaders is growing. The innate challenges of aid work, combined with the daunting political, technical, and security know-how required for these efforts, necessitates well-trained leaders and responders who understand a rapidly changing environment. Advancing the training needed for the development of such an imposing skill set will require us to draw on such diverse disciplines as human rights, security, international law, and leadership skills.

These new humanitarian leaders will not be starting from a blank slate. The system of coordination for responders and humanitarian actors is here to stay. The "humanitarian architecture" is taking on new forms in places like Syria, and the final shape that the Cluster System will take is not clear. Thankfully, over the past few years, the aid community has shown an ability to create new ways to coordinate, new ways to share information, and new ways for competing organizations to collaborate in the field. Despite the steep demands of the aid environment, the humanitarian "architecture" has grown in flexibility and functionality, and will comprise the bulk of the response system for future crises.

On top of the work of coordination and professionalization, the aid community will have to grow in its responsiveness to donors and funders, turning some of its extensive data into clear metrics for progress. Governmental funders like USAID, the British Government's Department for International Development, and other agencies will require that emergency relief efforts achieve a measure of efficacy and hold the potential for long-term change. This transition in humanitarianism from simple emergency relief to sustainable development is an old goal, and one that has so far proven elusive. Even within organizations, relief activities are often siloed from developmental activities. There are no blueprints for translating the high-intensity, rapid-delivery programs of a relief setting into thoughtful and strategic long-term growth.

Another issue that will dominate the near-term future of aid is quality. The responses to the Haiti and the Ebola crises revealed the dangers of novice aid. Freshly minted NGOs will inevitably respond to future emergencies in similar ways, pushing into the field in an effort to make their name and providing aid solutions without a sense of professional accountability. These efforts will consume aid dollars and create little in the way of lasting, sustainable solutions—and sometimes not even adequate short-term solutions. This is not to say that there is no room for new organizations. Indeed, many of these groups can be far more nimble and provide a deeper and more sustained local investment than huge international NGOs. But these groups must do so with the recognition that there is a moral and ethical, as well as a practical, responsibility to provide quality assistance while being accountable to both recipients and donors.

A dominant feature of future aid will be the practical application of new technologies. The greatest drivers of recent change have been the mobile phone, social media, and increased access to information for both aid providers and aid recipients. Greater access to data should enhance innovation *and* accountability. The ability to share data, as illustrated by the KoBo Toolbox, or to gain new forms of intelligence, as shown by the Signal Program, are examples, but there are many other similar tools as well. Crowdsourced data, drone imagery, and the increasingly greater fluency of social media will make vital information available to everyone, including aid recipients, in close to real time. Blending, sifting, and rendering useful data, as well as maintaining transparency between aid providers and recipients, will make up a great deal of aid work in the future.

Finally, and probably most importantly, aid will move away from the concept of Western saviors who swoop in to fix the troubles of the world. The most effective aid is that which comes from within. Building the local and national capacity of communities, governments, and even militaries is and will be the most effective and most sustainable solution for disaster aid. This is, of course, not easy to accomplish in regions affected by war and political disintegration. In areas like Syria and the ISIS-controlled regions of the Middle East, local capacity building means investing in local relief organizations that have greater ability to gain access and provide a stable base of operations than external group.

The move toward localization of humanitarian aid has a thorny side. The aid world is increasingly populated by newer actors that work in very different ways than traditional aid agencies. These new actors include not only local organizations, but also private industry and those with an interest in economic recovery. As other nations see participation in humanitarian responses as a vehicle for promoting their own national interests, the aid world will become further crowded. The challenges to the UN coordination system and the traditional aid actors will become greater as new government aid providers from the United States, China, Russia, India, and Middle Eastern nations enter the maelstrom of humanitarian aid. These newer actors are less likely to ascribe to some basic principles of humanitarianism like neutrality, independence, and impartiality, either because they are naïve or because they are profiteering. They are more likely to provide aid in a way geared toward furthering their own political objectives, a shift that deals a direct blow to the foundations of "neutral" humanitarian assistance.

The pessimistic view of these future changes in the humanitarian aid world is that they will lead to an unraveling of coordination and a disintegration of the basic principles of humanitarianism and human rights generated by the formation of the International Red Cross movement and the Geneva Conventions. In this gloomy scenario, organizations, militaries, and individual actors will work independently and largely with a view to their own best interests in delivering aid.

I have a more hopeful view of the future. I foresee the potential for an aid world where there are robust ways to educate, include, monitor, and promote new aid agencies, building on the lessons of the past and employing the best tools for coordination and a heightened sense of accountability to those we serve. This improved version of humanitarianism will certainly not come about by default or by accident, but will require new and creative engagements with the existing giants of aid.

In the future, I imagine myself in the back of a classroom in Amman, Jordan, watching the instructor move through a multimedia case study on the history of the Syrian conflict. The teacher's theme is protection of healthcare workers in war. Students from Iran, Pakistan, Turkey, the United States, and Europe all open their laptops as a Skype call comes up on the screen. A coordinator with experience in the most recent humanitarian emergency drops in via videoconference to discuss the challenges of access and the work of the health cluster. The students ask questions about their upcoming field internships, in which they will be paired with leaders to better understand how to guide an organization in the midst of a crisis response.

The classroom conversation turns to what can be learned from past responses, and a student asks me about my own field experience. In answering their questions, I try to give them a sense of how far the aid world has come since I first started practicing in it, including some of my own mistakes that I have made over the years. I also try to explain how they, as future leaders, can build on the work of the preceding generation of humanitarians—a form of professional humility. Indeed, as I continue my career with one foot in the medical world and the other in the humanitarian world, the most important sentiment that I've come away with is humility. The crises of the world are immensely complex, and humanitarian assistance will never be a perfect solution. We should, however, strive to make it a better one.

It has been a significant and difficult adjustment to move away from field work and toward the work of mentoring and teaching. The immediate care of my patients, whether in the emergency department or in the field, is still the single most powerful motivator for excellence. I still practice as a clinician in the emergency room, but where I once rushed into the field for every crisis, I now watch my students and colleagues take the lead in the responses to Syria's civil war and West Africa's Ebola epidemic—as I will in the next international crisis to arise.

When I look back on my career, I expect that its greatest impact will reside not in the lives of those patients I've helped directly, the new research I've explored, or even the hospitals I've helped build, but in the contributions of my students and trainees. Seeing the humanitarians I have taught practice medicine, organize relief efforts, and in turn teach yet another generation of aid workers is the most worthwhile legacy I can imagine. As more and more students pursue careers in global health, there will be a boom in humanitarian leadership. I feel a sense of responsibility to these future humanitarians. I owe it to them to teach them well, for their own understanding and for the lives they will touch. Like me, they will probably learn best from their mistakes.

Stepping back from the field and seeing my students take on new leadership roles has prompted me to reflect on my own motivations. I again recall William Osler's discourse on "Aequanimitas," encouraging future physicians to become objective and dispassionate in their approach to patients. More than a century later, Osler's equanimity showed me a way to help the rapidly expanding aid world. The infusion of science into this complex and dynamic pursuit can create a better, more predictable way of helping people affected by crisis. But the original motive—empathy—that brought me into medicine in the first place, and which motivates thousands of new humanitarians to head to the field and take very real risks, cannot be underemphasized. The humanitarian field will always be driven by empathic compassion, and not solely by scientific reasoning. Ultimately, I think that these two competing motivators, equanimity and empathy, can guide the future humanitarian. The leaders of the next generation of aid will ideally care deeply for the plight of those in need and will also understand the need to measure, optimize, and professionalize.

War, disaster, and displacement will always be with us, as will the principles upon which modern humanitarianism was built. Despite changes and challenges, we must carry these principles forward into the future and keep the "human" in humanitarian. Reflecting on a life in humanitarian medicine, and my own evolution from physician to researcher to teacher, I feel both privileged and responsible: it has been a privilege to participate in an evolving field, and I feel responsible, along with my peers, for training and advancing the next generation. Future humanitarians are our best hope, and investing in your best hope makes a profound kind of sense.

AFTERWORD

WITH HUNDREDS OF THOUSANDS OF REFUGEES PRESS-
ing on its borders, Europe is facing the worst refugee crisis since the
Second World War. The expansion of the regional refugee crisis in the
Middle East has become an increasing global issue. The sheer numbers of refugees seeking safety are staggering. The United Nations
High Commissioner for Refugees (UNHCR) estimates that at present
nearly 60 million people—the highest-ever estimate of the global refugee population—have been forcibly displaced by conflict and political
instability. Nearly 20 million are true refugees, having crossed an international border to escape persecution. Many are smuggled by boat,
train, or truck across Turkey, Serbia, and Hungary to claim asylum in
Germany, Sweden, Italy, and Austria.

Unbearable images of drowned Syrian children on the shores of
Turkey and migrants suffocated in a truck on an Austrian highway
compel us to consider what we stand for in the defense of the rights of
refugees fleeing persecution. The salient events of the refugee crisis have
galvanized citizens of Europe and Western nations, but they also have
created a deep divide among nations struggling to accommodate the

next wave of refugees and have led to a further schism within nations, as citizens are increasingly opposed to the resettlement of asylum seekers.

With such a massive wave of migrants moving toward European borders, the very foundations of European human rights principles have been shaken. The obligations required by international law have been challenged as nations are faced with hundreds of thousands, even millions, of refugees. Indeed, borders previously open to refugees and asylum seekers are increasingly closed as greater and greater numbers of refugees arrive. Even dangerous and highly publicized sea rescues by European aid organizations are seen by governments as encouraging greater numbers of refugees to face the risks to gain asylum.

The global humanitarian community must once again adapt itself to working in a new operating environment, namely European countries typically considered too developed to face such crises. Established humanitarian aid providers must operate within the complexities of shifting refugee policies and intense political pressures and contend with hundreds of new, grassroots efforts to assist displaced populations. We face a humanitarian emergency requiring rapid, stabilizing assistance as well as a political emergency requiring unified leadership. But the European response has been exceptionally fragmented, leaving aid agencies without a clear vision of what they can do to assist. Many humanitarians feel that the responses to the refugee crisis should be governed by the international laws set forth after World War II and assisted by the UNHCR. We have empowered the UNHCR to address refugee crises for the past five decades and must allow the same principles that have driven the response to refugees from Sudan into Kenya, from Rwanda into Tanzania, and from Kosovo into Albania.

But the present problem is not at all straightforward. The current refugee crisis has evolved from local and regional displacement to a global flow of refugees that can overwhelm host nations. Many fear that the migration could precipitate economic and political destabilization throughout the European Union. The unprecedented flow of refugees and internally displaced persons has created large pockets of instability, economic tensions, and xenophobia. Eventually the consequences of the crisis could erode political support for the core provisions of the 1951 UN Refugee Convention itself.

As we contemplate yet another challenge to the humanitarian community, it is useful to recount the values that underpin our industry. The French philosopher François Jean, who helped guide Médecins Sans Frontières, remarked:

> Humanitarian aid aims to preserve life in dignity and respect; it attempts to deliver aid in a time of crisis and to give back to people their capacity for choice. Respect for human dignity is at times not too compatible with mass-oriented operations. The "assisted populations" and "vulnerable groups" frequently referenced in the jargon of relief workers are not, it must be remembered, clusters of physiological organisms. Humanitarian action has nothing to do with some sort of veterinary compassion. The concern for others that guides us is applied to human beings, not to digestive apparatuses.[1]

Once again, the humanitarian community must revisit the core tenets of humanity—neutrality, impartiality, and independence—and determine how to best navigate this most recent challenge to humanitarianism. The future of millions will depend on how we learn, adapt and respond.

NOTES

CHAPTER 2: FIRST STEPS

1. Michael Buerk, "Extent of Ethiopia Famine Revealed," BBC News, October 23, 1984.
2. Charles Clements, *Witness to War* (New York: Bantam Books, 1984).
3. Graham Hancock, *The Lords of Poverty: the Power, Prestige and Corruption of the International Aid Business* (New York: Atlantic Monthly Press, 1989).
4. Liane Hansen, "Arms Overflow in Markets of Somalia," *Sunnikhalid* (Weekend Edition Sunday), January 3, 1993.

CHAPTER 3: CAREER HUMANITARIAN

1. Richard Grant and Julia Nijman, "Foreign Aid in the 1990s: Crisis or Transition?" *Tijdschrift voor economische en sociale geografie (TESG; Journal of Economic and Social Geography)* 86, no. 3 (June 1995): 215–218.

CHAPTER 4: GROWING CHALLENGES

1. Tania Bryer, interview with Bill Clinton, "We Could Have Saved 300,000 Lives in Rwanda," *CNBC Meets,* March 13, 2013.
2. John Borton, "Joint Evaluation of Emergency Assistance to Rwanda: Overseas Development Institute," London, June 1996.
3. Steve Inskeep, interview with Madeleine Albright, "Albright: U.N. Needs To Show Its Relevance On Syrian Issue," NPR, September 26, 2013.

CHAPTER 5: IN THE FIELD

1. Jennifer Clapp, *Hunger in the Balance: The New Politics of International Food Aid* (New York: Cornell University Press, 2012).

CHAPTER 6: FINDING HUMANITARIAN SPACE

1. Richard Horton, "Health in the Occupied Palestinian Territory 2011," *Lancet,* July 5, 2011.
2. G. Burnham, "Mortality After the 2003 Invasion of Iraq: A Cross-Sectional Cluster Sample Survey," *Lancet* 368, no. 9545 (October 21, 2006): 1421–1428.

CHAPTER 7: A NEW ERA OF CHALLENGES

1. Ian Fischer, "Chaos in Congo: A Primer. Many Armies Ravage Rich Land in the 'First World War' of Africa," *New York Times,* February 6, 2000.
2. BBC World Service, "Denis Mukwege: The Rape Surgeon of DRC," interview for *Outlook, BBC Magazine,* February 19, 2013.
3. Transcript, "Presentation to the United Nations 25/9/2012 by Dr. Denis Mukwege," Panzi Hospital, October 9, 2012, http://www.panzihospital.org/archives /1027 (retrieved October 22, 2014).

CHAPTER 8: PROTECTING HUMANITARIAN MEDICINE

1. Andrew Bostrom, *Human Rights Violations in the Syrian Health System: Perceptions, Beliefs, and Attitudes about Justice and Accountability Physicians for Human Rights Report,* 2015.
2. "Health Care in Danger: Violent Incidents Affecting Health Care, January to December 2012," International Committee of the Red Cross, 2013.

AFTERWORD

1. This is from a collection of essays by François Jean (1956–1999): Kevin P. Q. Phelan, ed., *From Ethiopia to Chechnya: Reflections on Humanitarian Action, 1988–1999,* trans. Richard Swanson (Doctors Without Borders/Médecins Sans Frontières, 2008).

RESOURCES

I have provided few specific references throughout the book, but there is, of course, much more detail to be learned about the evolution of modern humanitarianism. From field trade guides like the Sphere Handbook to new references to the humanitarian architecture, there are some important readings to add detail to the topics that, for the sake of brevity, I have covered superficially. In addition, the HHI team has produced and compiled some excellent and succinct resources for understanding the nuances of the international humanitarian architecture. For far more detail on current humanitarian practice, you might find some of these web resources helpful:

References and resources for the Harvard Humanitarian Initiative: www.hhi
.harvard.edu
The USAID Office of Foreign Disaster Assistance e-learning on the Humanitarian
Architecture, produced by HHI: www.buildingabetterresponse.com
The Advanced Training in Humanitarian Action on line learning portal: www
.atha.se
For current resources regarding aid in crisis, go to: www.reliefweb.org
The United Nations High Commission for Refugees: www.unhcr.org

THE HUMANITARIAN ARCHITECTURE

"Guidance for Humanitarian Country Teams." Geneva: Inter-Agency Standing Committee, 2009. https://www.humanitarianresponse.info/system/files/documents/files/IASC%20Guidance%20for%20Humanitarian%20Country%20Teams%2C%20Nov%2009.pdf.
"Guidance Note on Using the Cluster Approach to Strengthen Humanitarian Response." Geneva: Inter-Agency Standing Committee, 2009. http://www.who.int/hac/network/interagency/news/iastc_guidance_note.pdf?ua=1.
Handbook for RCs and HCs on Emergency Preparedness and Response. Geneva: Inter-Agency Standing Committee, 2010. http://interagencystandingcommittee.org/node/2867.

"International Humanitarian Architecture." *Disaster Response in Asia and the Pacific.* United Nations, 2015. http://www.unocha.org/publications/asiadisasterresponse /InternationalHumanitarianArchitecture.html.

"OCHA on Message: Inter-Agency Standing Committee." United Nations, 2012. https://docs.unocha.org/sites/dms/Documents/120229_OOM-IASC_eng.pdf.

Walker, P., and D. Maxwell. *Shaping the Humanitarian World.* UK: Routledge, 2008.

OCHA REFERENCES, AND
REFERENCE TO THE BBR COURSE

Building a Better Response E-Learning Course. http://www.buildingabetterrespo nse.org/.

"Coordination to Save Lives: History and Emerging Challenges," *Policies and Studies Series.* United Nations, 2012. https://docs.unocha.org/sites/dms/Documents /Coordination%20to%20Save%20Lives%20History%20and%20Emerging %20Challenges.pdf.

"OCHA on Message: Humanitarian Principles." United Nations, 2012. https://docs .unocha.org/sites/dms/Documents/OOM-humanitarianprinciples_eng_June 12.pdf.

This is OCHA. New York: United Nations, 2012. https://docs.unocha.org/sites/dms/ Documents/OCHA_Brochure_Eng_2012.pdf.

HUMAN RIGHTS AND HUMAN RIGHTS LAW

Englebert, Pierre, and Denis M. Tull. "Postconflict Reconstruction in Africa: Flawed Ideas about Failed States." *International Security* 32, no. 4 (2008): 106–139.

Geneva Conventions. ICRC. https://www.icrc.org/en/war-and-law/treaties-customary -law/geneva-conventions.

The Geneva Conventions of 12 August 1949. ICRC. https://www.icrc.org/eng/assets /files/publications/icrc-002-0173.pdf.

Paris, Roland. "Saving Liberal Peacebuilding." *Review of International Studies* 36, no. 2 (2010): 337–365.

Tull, Denis M. "Peacekeeping in the Democratic Republic of Congo: Waging Peace and Fighting War." *International Peacekeeping* 16, no. 2 (2009): 215–230.

Universal Declaration of Human Rights. United Nations. http://www.un.org/en/docu ments/udhr/.

Vinck P., and P. N. Pham. "Searching for Lasting Peace: Population-Based Survey on Perceptions and Attitudes about Peace, Security and Justice in Eastern Democratic Republic of the Congo." Harvard Humanitarian Initiative, United Nations Development Programme, 2014. www.peacebuildingdata.org/drc.

INTERNATIONAL HUMANITARIAN LAW

Bergholm, Linnea. "The African Union, the United Nations and Civilian Protection Challenges in Darfur." *Refugee Studies Centre Working Paper Series,* no. 63, May 2010. http://www.rsc.ox.ac.uk/PDFs/RSCworkingpaper63.pdf.

Bouchet-Saulnier, Francoise. "Introduction to International Humanitarian Law," Crimes of War Project, November 2007. http://www.crimesofwar.org/thebook /intro-ihl.html.

Bouchet-Saulnier, Francoise. *The Practical Guide to Humanitarian Law.* Lanham, MD: Rowman & Littlefield, 2014.

"Cross-Cutting Report: Protection of Civilians in Armed Conflict." Security Council Report, no. 4, October 2009. http://www.securitycouncilreport.org/cross-cutting -report/protection-of-civilians-in-armed-conflict-1.php.

Dinstein, Yoram. "The Right to Humanitarian Assistance." *Naval War College Review* (Autumn 2000): 77–91. http://ihl.ihlresearch.org/index.cfm?fuseaction=page.vi ewPage&pageID=808&nodeID=2.

Dubois, Marc. "Civilian Protection and Humanitarian Advocacy: Strategies and (False?) Dilemmas." *Humanitarian Exchange Magazine* issue 39 (June 2008). http://www.odihpn.org/report.asp?id=2917.

HPCR, "60 Years of the Geneva Conventions: The Role of International Law in Protecting Civilians," web seminar, Program on Humanitarian Policy and Conflict Research at Harvard, August 2009. http://www.hpcrresearch.org/events/60 -years-geneva-conventions-role-international-law-protecting-civilians.

International Humanitarian Law Distance Learning Series. Advanced Training Program on Humanitarian Action. http://www.atha.se/elearning.

Maogoto, Jackson Nyamuya, and Gywnn MacCarrick. "Typology of Conflict: Terrorism and the Ambiguation of the Laws of War." *GNLU Law Review* 2, no. 1 (February 26, 2010).

HUMANITARIAN OPERATIONAL GUIDANCE

Bolton P., and J. Bass, L. Murray, K. Lee, W. Weiss, S. M. McDonnell. "Expanding the Scope of Humanitarian Program Evaluation." *Prehospital and Disaster Medicine* 22, no. 5 (December 2007): 390–395.

Pham P. N., and P. Vinck. "Technology, Conflict Early Warning Systems, Public Health, and Human Rights." *Health and Human Rights* 14, no. 2 (December 2012): 2–12.

Walker, Peter and Catherine Russ. "Professionalising the Humanitarian Sector: A Scoping Study." Enhancing Learning & Research for Humanitarian Assistance, April 2010.

Wassenhove, Van. "L.N. Blackett Memorial Lecture: Humanitarian Aid Logistics: Supply Chain Management in High Gear." *Journal of the Operational Research Society* 57 (2006): 475–489.

URBANIZATION AND HUMANITARIAN CRISIS

Active Learning Network for Accountability and Performance in Humanitarian Action. http://www.alnap.org/resources/lessons.aspx.

Patel R., and T. Burke. "Urbanization: An Emerging Humanitarian Disaster." *New England Journal of Medicine* 361, no. 8 (August 2009): 741–743.

Sanderson, D., Clarke P. Knox, and L. Campbell. "Responding to Urban Disasters: Learning from Previous Relief and Recovery Operations." ALNAP, November 2012.

Schoeller-Diaz, David Alejandro, and Victoria_Alicia López, John Joseph "Ian" Kelly IV, and Ronak B. Patel. "Hope in the Face of Displacement and Rapid Urbanization." *HHI Working Paper Series,* September 2012.

CIVIL-MILITARY HUMANITARIAN ISSUES

"Guidelines on the Use of Foreign Military and Civil Defense. Assets in Disaster Relief–Oslo Guidelines.'" United Nations Rev. 1.1, November 2007.

Metcalfe, Victoria, Simone Haysom, and Stuart Gordon. "Trends and Challenges in Humanitarian Civil-Military Coordination. A Review of the Literature." *HPG Working Paper,* May 2012.

Wiharta, Sharon, Hassan Ahmad, Jean-Yves Haine, Josefina Löfgren, and Tim Randall. "The Effectiveness of Foreign Military Assets in Natural Disaster Response." Stockholm International Peace Research Institute, 2008.

SPHERE HUMANITARIAN STANDARDS

Darcy, James. "Locating Responsibility: The Sphere Humanitarian Charter and its Rationale from Disasters." *Disasters* 28, no. 2 (June 2004): 112–123.

Sphere Handbook in Action E-learning Course. The Sphere Project. http://www.sphere project.org/learning/e-learning-course/.

The Sphere Handbook 2011: Humanitarian Charter and Standards in Humanitarian Response. The Sphere Project, 2011. http://www.sphereproject.org/content /view/720/200/lang,english.

Tong, Jacqui. "Questionable Accountability: MSF and Sphere in 2003." *Disasters* 28, no. 2 (2004): 176–189.

Walker, P., and S. Purdin. "Birthing Sphere. The Early History of the Sphere Project." *Disasters* 28, no. 2 (June 2004): 100–111.

CRITICISMS AND COMMENTARIES

Ferris, E. "Faith Based and Secular Humanitarian Organizations." *International Review of the Red Cross* 87, no. 858 (June 2005): 311–325.

Hilhorst, D. "Being Good at Doing Good? Quality and Accountability of Humanitarian NGOs." *Disasters* 26, no. 3 (2002): 193–212.

Roberts L., and M. VanRooyen. "Ensuring Public Health Neutrality." *New England Journal of Medicine* 368 (March 21, 2013): 1073–1075. http://www.nejm.org /doi/full/10.1056/NEJMp1300197.

Terry, Fiona. *Condemned to Repeat? The Paradox of Humanitarian Action.* Ithaca, NY: Cornell University Press, 2002.

"United States Agency for International Development: Working with Faith Based Organizations. Bush Brings Faith to Foreign Aid: As Funding Rises, Christian Groups Deliver Help—With a Message." *Boston Globe,* October 8, 2006.

INDEX

199

ABOUT THE AUTHOR

MICHAEL VANROOYEN, MD, MPH, IS THE DIRECTOR OF the Harvard Humanitarian Initiative (HHI) at Harvard University and the Chairman of Emergency Medicine at Brigham and Women's Hospital in Boston.

Dr. VanRooyen has worked as an emergency physician with numerous relief organizations in over thirty countries affected by war and disaster, including Somalia, Bosnia, Rwanda, Iraq, North Korea, Darfur-Sudan, Chad, and the Democratic Republic of the Congo. He has worked in the field as a relief expert with several nongovernmental organizations and has been a policy advisor to several UN organizations and is a member of the Inter-Agency Standing Committee Health Cluster. He also serves on the Board of Overseers for the International Rescue Committee. He has testified before Congress and at numerous UN briefings on policy issues related to Iraq, Darfur, and the Democratic Republic of the Congo and served on a National Academies/GAO review of mortality in Darfur.

Domestically, Dr. VanRooyen worked with the American Red Cross to provide relief assistance at the site of the World Trade Center in New York on September 11, 2001. He also helped to coordinate the American Red Cross public health response to Hurricane Katrina and has worked as a physician with the US Secret Service, NASA, and with the US Public Health Service with the Navajo and Apache tribes in Arizona and New Mexico, respectively.

Dr. VanRooyen is a Professor at Harvard Medical School and the Harvard School of Public Health, where he teaches courses on humanitarian operations in war and disaster. In 2012, he founded the Humanitarian Academy at Harvard, an educational program to advance humanitarian professionalism.

He lives in Wayland, Massachusetts, with his wife, Julia VanRooyen, MD, and their three children, Alexandra, Jackson, and Isabella.